Rehabilitation for MCI and Dementia:

Using Assistive Technology to Support Daily Activities

May this book help regain, increase, and maintain the smiles of people with MCI/dementia and their families

Rehabilitation for MCI and Dementia:

Using Assistive Technology to Support Daily Activities

Kiyoshi Yasuda, Ph.D.

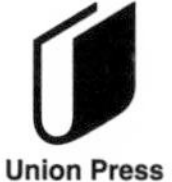

Union Press

First published 2022
by Union Press®
(a division of Union Services Co., Ltd.)
1-6, Uehommachi-Nishi 5 chome, Chuo-ku, Osaka, 542-0062 Japan
www.union-services.com

DTP by Design International
Printed and bound by Shinano Co., Ltd.

ISBN 978-4-909848-13-0

Printed in Japan

This work was supported by JSPS KAKENHI Grant-in-Aid for Publication of Scientific Research Results (Grant Number 20HP6003).

Foreword

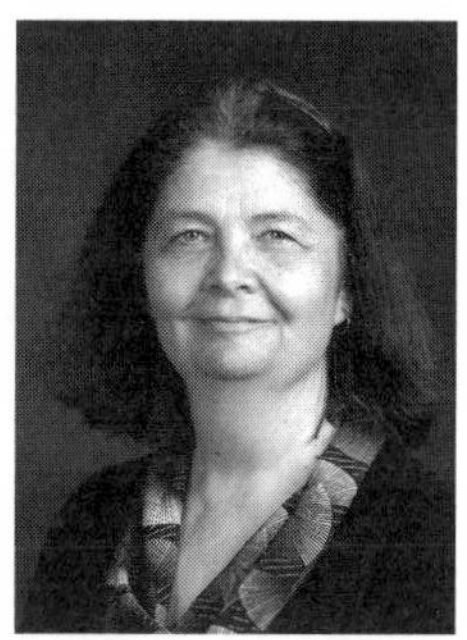

In the 1990's, on opposite sides of the globe, two speech-language pathologists were challenged to help persons with memory problems find solutions due to dementia. Prof. Yasuda in Japan and myself in the U.S.A. developed a similar, and practical, approach to supporting word retrieval difficulties: external memory aids. In our own unique ways, we both developed tools for providing written cues that would allow the person to maintain their conversational and functional skills, from memory books and reminder cards to written notes and auditory messages. We both created clothing and devices to ensure that the person would have their memory aid with them when needed. We finally met each other in 2008 when I was awarded a Fellowship by the Japan Society for the Advancement of Science and spent several months at the Prefectural University of Hiroshima. We have shared ideas, books, and advice ever since.

I was honored when Prof. Yasuda asked me to review the English translation of this book. It was a pleasure to learn, in more detail, about his very clever memory aid devices and the research studies he conducted to confirm their effectiveness. Prof. Yasuda has been working tirelessly over the past decades to support persons with dementia and their family members in multiple ways. With the understanding that it may take many more years before medical science truly understands the causes of dementia and develops effective medicines to prevent or cure it, Prof. Yasuda advocates for a continuum of services and resources to care for these persons with dementia.

First, he describes the necessity of obtaining a thorough diagnostic evaluation to best understand the range and diversity of presenting symptoms. He explains persons' changing needs as the disease takes its degenerative course, and organizes the supportive tools using a stage model, from mild to moderate to severe dementia. The services of the Memory Clinic at the Chiba Rosai Hospital are described, as well as other resources such as the national insurance plan. Most of the chapters of this book detail the many different types of assistive technology, for each stage of dementia, including the more recent development of internet-based tools. The New Memory Support Diary for persons with mild memory loss and the various wearable adaptations are examples of Low-Tech AT that give them confidence to manage their memory concerns independently. The IC Recorder developed for persons at moderate stage is a versatile Middle-Tech reminding tool that has many practical everyday applications. His most clever AT for persons with mild/moderate dementia is the High-Tech *anime* grandchild agent who serves as a conversation partner and motivation to accomplish desired tasks. He recognizes, however, that without a network of education and technical assistance in using and adapting these tools to individual circumstances, persons and their families may not maximize their use of this technology. His examples of workshops, educational programs, and support groups will serve as models for others interested in promoting these services.

It is laudable that Prof. Yasuda acknowledges the importance of families, friends, and professional caregivers in supporting the everyday activities of persons with dementia. He provides multiple examples of technology to enable interpersonal interactions among persons, and to oversee the safety of persons with dementia living alone. He recommends support groups for sharing ideas and problem -solving difficulties encountered by families. His advocacy for government-supported assistance extends from assistive technology lending centers to home safety equipment and financial incentives for volunteers.

This book is not just a compendium of useful assistive technologies, it is a complete and model program for the care and support of persons with dementia and their families. To clinicians, administrators, families, and anyone else who is interested in helping persons with dementia, I wholeheartedly recommend this book to you. Prof. Yasuda's expertise and creativity in improving the lives of persons with dementia is a gift to us all.

Michelle S. Bourgeois, Ph.D., CCC-SLP
Tampa, Florida, U.S.A.

Preface

The main symptom of MCI (Mild Cognitive Impairment), as well as of dementia, is memory disturbance. The training of persons with memory disturbance is accompanied by difficulties that they easily forget what they have just memorized. In particular, as dementia is progressive, the effect of training is limited. For a person with impaired visual acuity, hearing impairment, or gait disturbance, we encourage them to live an independent life by having them use a pair of glasses, a hearing aid, or a wheelchair. Thus, we should also support the life of persons with MCI or dementia by using memory aids. Even professionals in the field, however, often either do not have or do not think of such an idea.

I began to work at Chiba Rosai Hospital in 1983 as a speech-language pathologist, and was given opportunities to work with persons who were suffering from memory impairments developed after brain injuries. I looked for memory aids for these persons but found few such aids, and as a result decided to try to produce them for the persons. Since around 1993, persons with dementia began to come to our rehabilitation department seeking evaluation and training. At first, I attempted to give them paper drills of arithmetic and of *kanji* characters known later as "brain-training," but the stage of dementia of some persons was clearly getting worse. Therefore, I experimentally applied some memory aids and eventually observed positive reactions from the persons. Since then, I have strived to develop new memory aids. IC (integrated circuit) recorders and other ICT (information and communication technology) devices available on the market were also utilized to support the daily lives of persons with MCI and dementia.

In 1997, Dr. Tadashi Misu at Chiba Institute of Technology and I created a Voice-Output Memory-Aid. Since then, I have been involved in collaborative studies with universities of engineering and research institutes on how to support the daily lives of persons with MCI and dementia by using videophones, action recognition, virtual agents and other high-technology systems. Currently, I am affiliated with Osaka Institute of Technology and Kyoto Prefectural University of Medicine. I have also proposed an idea for using dogs which carry ICT devices and tools to support their owner who is suffering from dementia.

Memory aids are traditionally called compensatory aids, external memory aids, supportive devices, welfare devices, etc. They are grouped into the term "Assistive Technology (AT)" which in this book includes software applications and various therapeutic approaches. Among them, memo-pads, diaries, and other products without electric power supply were categorized as low-technology AT, (Low-Tech AT). Commercially available ICT devices and other electronic products were categorized as middle-technology AT (Middle-Tech AT). Experimental products and systems which are being studied in universities and research institutes were categorized as high-technology AT (High-Tech AT). We need Low-Tech AT because we cannot support every aspect of the daily lives of persons with dementia only by using Middle-Tech AT and High-Tech AT, or AI (Artificial Intelligence) that it is currently receiving remarkable attention.

This book introduces ATs that could be used to support home dwelling persons with dementia, and it also illustrates practical examples that make use of these ATs. Many of the Low-Tech ATs introduced in Chapters 2 and 5 were in fact developed by myself, because there had been few practical ATs which could be applied to persons with MCI and mild/moderate dementia. For persons with severe dementia, memory and communication aids were introduced in Bourgeois (2014).

In most of the widely accepted textbooks, reflective attitudes, or redirection techniques have been recommended for dementia caring. For example, "Let's look for it together" when the person with dementia insists that his/her belonging is missing or stolen, and "Let's go together" when the person tries to go out alone. Reflective attitudes, or redirection techniques, however, do not always work depending upon the situations and the family member's attitude. Fortunately, devices are now available on the market for searching for one's belongings and a lost person. Such devices and possible Middle-Tech ATs are presented in Chapters 3, 4, 5 and 6. Various trials using High-Tech AT are introduced in Chapter 7.

In Chapter 1, I will explain memory disturbances and screening methods for MCI and dementia and evaluate "prevention theories" of dementia. In Chapter 8, rehabilitation approaches at a memory clinic and self/mutual/social supports are demonstrated. In the appendices, readers can find useful resources such as lists of memory strategies for the healthy elderly.

This book is aimed mainly at rehabilitation staff working in memory clinics who support persons with MCI or dementia dwelling at home. I also expect that this book will be utilized by the following people for the following purposes: care staff in the elderly facilities to apply ATs, people who love handicraft to create Low-Tech ATs, people who are familiar with a wide range of ICT appliances to discover new Middle-Tech ATs, programmers to develop more useful software applications, engineers to research High-Tech ATs, persons with MCI or dementia and their family members to evaluate usability of ATs and propose issues that they want to resolve with AT, administrative officials to start AT lending services, and volunteers to open "AT cafés" where AT users can receive advice on using ATs. I would like to call these people "professionals" in this field.

The contents of this book place an emphasis on introductions of various ATs and of actual cases who adopted ATs. There are many books that explain the traditional approaches for coping with dementia. In recent years, several books on dementia and AT have also been published which are listed in the references. Readers are first advised to read these books, then to study this book as one of the new supplementary methods to such approaches.

Japanese references and products are often cited in this book. If you copy and paste PDF files of the references or URLs of the producing companies to free translation services, such as DeepL Translator or Google Translate, you can easily translate them into various languages.

Dementia is unfortunately incurable in the current medical field. However, if you can utilize available ATs to the fullest extent, it is possible for persons with MCI or dementia to maintain their QOL, to prolong the period of their independent lives, and to participate in social activities. I hope that professionals in the field will make the effort to develop more efficient ATs and interventions while sharing experiences of success and failure, in order to support their daily lives.

Acknowledgments

I would like to express my deepest gratitude to Dr. Noriko Nagatsuka and Dr. Michelle S. Bourgeois. Without their help in checking the English translation, it would have been impossible for me to complete this book.

To produce this book I have received much support from persons with MCI/dementia, their families, professional caregivers, volunteers, students, and researchers at universities and institutions, staff members at Chiba Rosai Hospital and its headquarters, and my family members.

I also appreciate ESCOR Co., Ltd., the publisher of the original Japanese version of this book. For the last five years, Union Press has inspired me to continue to write this book in English.

This book has been completed after many trials and failures over 35 years, with the help and encouragement from the many people mentioned above.

Finally, I dedicate this book to my parents, who taught me the importance of rehabilitation, alternative aids, and even QOL at the time when the concepts and the words "rehabilitation" and "QOL" were not known to society.

Contents

CHAPTER ONE

Memory, assessment for MCI/dementia, and rehabilitation

1. Types of memory and memory impairment

The primary symptom of MCI (Mild Cognitive Impairment) and dementia is memory impairment. Chapter 1 begins with explaining about memory and memory impairment. Experiences and knowledge that people have accumulated in the course of life are categorized into various types of memory and are saved in the brain so that you can recall them easily. According to Baddeley (1995), memory consists mainly of procedural memory, sensory memory, working memory, episodic memory, and semantic memory (see Hickey & Bourgeois (2018) for details).

1.1 Procedural memory

Procedural memory is the kind of memory that people learn using their bodies, such as swimming or driving. Procedural memory is associated deeply with the cerebellum, and it tends not to be lost easily and is often relatively preserved until the last stage of dementia. Persons with dementia may say that they "have forgotten how to use the tool," yet they often recall the way to use it once they hold the tool, as the old saying "he is an old hand at it" goes.

1.2 Sensory memory

Sensory memory is the short term storage of information that arrives directly from our senses (i.e., hearing, vision, touch, taste, and smell). Vestibular and somatosensory stimuli (i.e., pain, temperature, and proprioception) also enter sensory memory. Information is transferred to working memory and even to episodic or semantic memory.

1.3 Working memory

Various information enters our brain through our senses and is held briefly in sensory memory for several seconds. Then it is held temporarily in working memory while being actively manipulated, although the working memory has a limited-capacity (see Mahendra, Hickey, & Bourgeois, 2018, for details). In everyday life, we often use multiple kinds of memory functions at the same time. For example, we need to remember a telephone number until we finish entering it. While we are looking at an old photo album, we need to remember to take medicines when the time comes. In remembering multiple actions, the function you simultaneously carry out is called "working memory." When you are cleaning the house while heating a pan in the kitchen and the bottom of a pot burns, this may be due to the impairment of working memory.

1.4 Episodic memory

Episodic memory is the kind of memory that a person actually experienced in the past. For example, people may remember the heat, smell, and sound of bombing they experienced during the war. This is a memory they experienced by using their five senses. On the other hand, knowledge about war obtained from watching TV, hearing from others, and reading books is called "semantic memory."

Episodic memory is also called autobiographical memory. It is the memory of where you were born, which schools you went to, what kinds of jobs you were engaged in, and other records of your life. It also includes the memory of what you ate for lunch, what you did last week, and other actions you undertook recently. Newly encoded episodic memory is kept in the hippocampus and its periphery located at the lower-inside of the brain. Thus, lesions in these areas cause anterograde amnesia or impairment of recent memory. The episodic memory resides in the hippocampus for sometime, then, moves to the parietal lobe or the inside of the parietal lobe. If you have a lesion or atrophy in these areas, you might forget the past experiences of several years, such as the company you worked for three years ago, or the fact that you lost your spouse five years ago. Most cases in Alzheimer's disease begin with episodic memory impairment. The episodic memory is further classified into several subtypes on the basis of temporal-context: anterograde memory, retrograde memory, recent memory, and remote memory.

1.5 Anterograde amnesia/Impairment of prospective memory

Imagine that a person had brain damage or developed dementia at some point in his/her life. Memory loss after the onset of the disease to the present is called "anterograde amnesia." In a severe case of anterograde amnesia, the person cannot remember any incidents after the onset of the illness. For instance, a 50-year-old person who developed anterograde amnesia at the age of 40 would not have accumulated any memories since the age of 40. The person might always answer, "I am 40 years old" to a questioner.

In many cases persons with dementia tend to develop anterograde amnesia in the first stage. They often fail to locate their wallet at the place they left it, and they often forget if they have already taken a medicine and try to take it again. People usually act according to their daily schedule; for example, "Tuesday is to go to the day-care center" or "June 1st is the day to see the doctor." However, it is especially hard for them to remember dates because the date changes every day. Memory of recalling a schedule is called "prospective memory," and anterograde amnesia often causes impairment of prospective memory as well. As a result, persons with anterograde amnesia have difficulties in living according to the schedule they have planned.

1.6 Retrograde amnesia

Some persons gradually lose the memories of incidents prior to the onset of their diseases. This type of amnesia is called "retrograde amnesia." As retrograde amnesia becomes more severe, the period of incidents they forget is further extended. For example, at the earlier stage they may not recall anything that happened for five years prior to the onset (5-year retrograde amnesia), and then gradually they forget most of the things that happened, for instance, in the last 20 years prior to the onset (20-year retrograde amnesia). There was a woman who developed retrograde amnesia in her 40s after a traffic accident and lost her memory as far back as 20 years prior to the accident. She had obtained a driver's license about 15 years before, yet she insisted, "I don't have a driver's license." This is because she lost her memory of the time when she obtained the license. She might have felt she was about 25 years old. This sort of past memory is also called remote episodic memory.

Another example is a couple who married five years ago. The husband developed retrograde amnesia and forgot anything that happened for seven or eight years prior to the onset. Thus, he forgot about his marriage and his wife. He would ask his wife, "You always take care of me kindly, but who are you?" He also suffered from anterograde amnesia, and so he could not remember anything although he was told every day who she was. Eventually, he started saying, "My girlfriend's name is Yoshiko." Yoshiko was his ex-girlfriend before he met his wife. In many cases, memories of persons with dementia go way back to old days. Their last remaining memory could be a remote episodic memory of their early childhood.

1.7 Semantic memory

Semantic memory is also known as "source memory." This type of memory is a collection of what people learned at school, watched on TV, read in books, and other knowledge people obtained from other people and the media. Semantic memory also includes knowledge of historical people, scientific facts, such as, Edison is an inventor, or the earth is round. This is the knowledge you obtained indirectly from sources such as textbooks and the news. However, if you actually met Edison, or saw the earth from space, these memories become your episodic memory. Therefore, whether the memory is a semantic memory or episodic one depends on the individual's experience. Persons at an early stage of Alzheimer's dementia forget what they ate for lunch just after they had it (episodic memory impairment), but they may be able to explain in detail about historical knowledge they have acquired by reading favorite books (semantic memory).

The type of memory that most animals have is considered to be episodic memory. Birds, for example, remember the places where they have hidden food, as episodic memory. Humans have developed languages, letters, radio, TV, and various other types of media. Consequently, I consider that we have come to have a much larger quantity of semantic memory than of episodic memory. There are various types of semantic memory, and some of them are described below by relating them to the corresponding episodic memory.

1.8 Memory of face

Memory of face is divided mainly into categories of family members and close acquaintances (episodic memory), and face memory of people who are well known on TV or in newspapers (semantic memory). An onset of retrograde amnesia would affect the episodic memory. At first, they are likely to forget the faces of people whom they have met recently. Then, they would forget in the following order: the faces of their grandchildren, and the faces of their sons' wives who have married several years ago. When the stage of dementia is progressed, the person might ask, "Who are you?" to his/her spouse. Or if a woman's son looks like her husband at a younger age, she would mistake her son for her husband.

If a person loses memory of the face of his/her favorite celebrity (semantic memory), he/she cannot recognize the face when seeing him/her on TV. For example, there was a person who was very fond of playing golf and failed to recognize the face of a famous golfer. Curiously enough, he was able to recognize the golfer by looking at him swinging a golf-club. This sometimes happens because memories of faces, actions, voices, and biographies of celebrity, etc. are stored in different areas respectively in the brain. However, when the stage of dementia becomes more severe, they forget not only faces but also the actions, biographies, etc.

1.9 Memory of geography and scenery

Knowledge about the locations of cities that you have never visited and well-known buildings, etc. are classified into semantic memory. When people can explain about the pyramids even though they have never been to Egypt, they are recollecting the knowledge from semantic memory. Meanwhile, memory of scenery where you live, or the exterior appearance of your house, is episodic memory. Episodic memories also include memory of directions, such as that of how to get to the toilet in your home and how to get to the station from your home. If you forget the exterior appearance of your house or toilet, you will get lost in town and your home. When persons with dementia visit their parents' home, for example, they often become uncomfortable. This is because they find the interior scene of their parents' house looks different from what they remember from the past.

1.10 Memory of objects

When people recognize objects, they need to match the object that they are actually seeing with the corresponding and prototypical memory of the object. If you lose your prototypical memory, you cannot recognize the object. People also cannot recognize newly produced objects because there are no prototypical memories for the object. For example, they cannot recognize a new type of toilet seat while they can recognize an old style one. Some persons with severe dementia may even eat a soap or frozen food when they have lost memories of the appearance as well as the smell or the temperature of it, which makes it difficult for them to judge whether it is edible or not. Some persons remember what "chopsticks" are (semantic memory) but they might not discern their chopsticks from those of family members due to their impairment of episodic memory.

Related Topics —Selective impairment of abstract knowledge—

Semantic memory includes memories of abstract knowledge, such as of the French Revolution, the Pythagorean theorem, and the division of the three powers of government. A woman who had an operation for a brain tumor recalled her past and her family (episodic memory). She could describe in detail the fact that she delivered a valedictorian speech as her academic performance was excellent, but memory tests revealed that she had lost considerable parts of abstract knowledge. During the tests, she told the examiner that, "I have never heard of the word *Meiji Ishin* (revolution), and of the name *Nobunaga Oda* (a famous Japanese historical figure)." When the atomic bomb was mentioned, she replied, "The atomic bomb? What is it?" Then, when an atomic bomb was explained to her, she said, "Oh, I know it, it was dropped near my home in Osaka (she meant a normal bomb not the atomic one in *Hiroshima* or *Nagasaki*)." In short, she lost a lot of abstract knowledge that she had learned. We hypothesized that abstract knowledge in semantic memory is related to the bilateral temporal lobes, especially the anterior half of the middle region of the left temporal lobe in the brain (Yasuda, Watanabe, & Ono, 1997). According to fMRI, when the names of friends (episodic memory) were presented, different areas of the brain were activated compared to when the names of famous people whom participants have never met (semantic memory) were given (Kawashima, 2003a).

1.11 Summary of memory impairments

Semantic memory is memories of information that everyone is supposed to share in society, and it is stored deeply in the temporal lobe. The temporal lobe, in fact, tends to atrophy in persons with Pick's disease. Consequently, their semantic memory deteriorates significantly. As a result, persons with

Pick's disease may develop social cognitive disorders and may behave in peculiar ways, such as not paying money when shopping, taking somebody's belongings without permission, and others. In contrast, persons with early stages of Alzheimer's disease would behave without violating social norms.

A person with Alzheimer's disease told his wife that, "I am going to Hawaii now" just after he watched a TV program about Hawaii. Another person said that, "A *sumo* wrestler is coming in the door" while watching *sumo* wrestling on TV. The contents of TV programs are to be categorized as semantic memory since people watch them through the media, but the difference between semantic memory and episodic memory becomes subtle for some persons and they may be confused.

To make it easier to understand the overview of memory impairments, the following figure (Yasuda, 2018) may be helpful. The orders of developing memory impairments are shown taking Alzheimer's disease as an example (Figure 1-1). Please also note that there are many other possible orders.

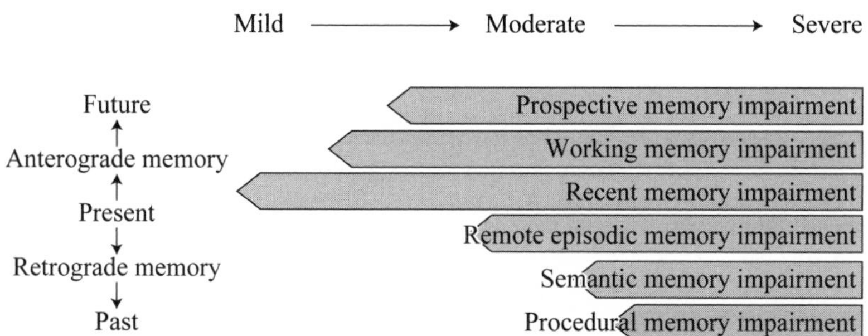

Figure 1-1 Orders of developing memory impairments

Related Topics —Why is it hard to recall people's names?—

The older we get, the harder it is to recall people's names. For the names of ordinary commodities (nouns), we are not allowed to name, for instance, "books" while pointing at "newspapers." This is because the linguistic meaning of what we call a "newspaper" is strictly defined. On the other hand, we can freely make a decision about people's names (proper names). For example, a slender person may have a name of *Futoshi* (meaning being fat). Thus, the proper name plays a role only to indicate the person, and it seldom relates to the meaning of the name. Therefore, it will be difficult to recall people's names based on their meanings. The proper name of "Mount *Fuji*" is often described as "the beautiful and the highest mountain in Japan." However, such descriptions are not the meanings of *Fuji*, but are the "attributes" of the mountain. The reason for this is that the height and appearance of *Fuji* could change if it should erupt. On the other hand, the meaning of "Mount" does not change.

We hypothesized that people's names are related to the fusiform gyrus and hippocampus on the inside of the left temporal lobe, and hypofunction of these areas caused by aging makes it harder for people to recall people's names (Yasuda, Nakamura, & Beckman, 2000a). The language centers are located in the cortex of the front-temporal-parietal lobes in the left hemisphere. Impairments in these areas cause aphasia. Persons with severe aphasia also cannot recall nouns and proper names. Although they have difficulties in understanding the meanings of nouns, they often understand the proper names. We hypothesized that the symptoms shown in severe aphasia are due to the difference between the meaning of the nouns and attributes of proper names (Yasuda et al., 2000). Subtypes of frontotemporal dementia sometimes develop from aphasia.

Bourgeois (1992) suggested that personally relevant single words remain spared into the moderate stages of Alzheimer's disease. She used personalized written cues for persons with moderate/severe dementia (Bourgeois, 2014). The written cues include proper names such as their family member's names and geographical names. Yasuda & Ono (1998) showed the well-preserved comprehension of famous personal names compared to nouns by persons with global aphasia. The comprehension of written personal names was more spared to those of verbally presented personal names. The preservation of written proper names by persons with dementia should be studied further.

2. Cognitive assessment for MCI and dementia

Selecting appropriate tests for assessment is important for the diagnosis of MCI (Petersen, Smith, Waring et al., 1999) and dementia. There are many persons with MCI and mild dementia who were once diagnosed as "memory is normal at their age." Such diagnoses were often based on the results obtained from a simple screening test such as the MMSE (Folstein, Folstein, & Mchugh, 1975). Early detection of disease helps persons prepare for learning coping methods for memory disturbances in addition to taking medications if needed. Chiba Rosai Hospital opened the Memory Clinic for outpatients at the Rehabilitation Department in 2004 (see Chapter 8). The purposes were the early detection of MCI and mild dementia and providing rehabilitation of daily-life support using Assistive Technology (AT). Although many kinds of criteria having been advocated for the diagnosis of MCI (Japanese Society of Neurology, 2017), the following section introduces the cognitive assessment battery used in the Memory Clinic of Chiba Rosai Hospital, as well as the results of the battery.

2.1 *Mini-Mental State Examination* (MMSE; Folstein et al., 1975)

MMSE is a screening test for dementia on a 30-point scale. People who score from 27 to 24 points are diagnosed with possible MCI, and people scoring 23 or under are diagnosed with possible dementia. There are many cases, however, in which people who obtained almost 30 points reveal low scores in the other cognitive assessments mentioned below. In fact, the underestimate for diagnoses of persons with MCI by the MMSE has been attributed to their simplified contents. Many biases exist in such a standardized test when the age, education, and cultural background of the individual assessed does not match the normative sample (Hickey, Khayum, & Bourgeois, 2018).

2.2 *Kana-hiroi (kana cancellation) test* (Kaneko, 1990)

This is a letter-cancellation test in which participants are to check five specified *kana* letters (Japanese phonograms) while reading a story written only in *kana*. The participant is required to carry out multi-tasks: remembering and cancelling five letters while silently reading the content. Thus, the divided attention test is aimed to measure working memory. Working memory is strongly associated with the frontal lobe of the brain (Kaneko, 1990). Participants with suspected frontal-lobe impairment sometimes show low scores on this test.

2.3 *Paired-associate learning test* (Related and unrelated-word pairs: Japan Society for Higher Brain Dysfunction, 2014)

Participants are required to memorize word pairs over three trials. At first, 10 sets of semantically-related word pairs such as "men-women" and "alcohol-beer" are verbally presented to the participant. Then, the examiner says the word "men" and the participant is to respond "women." The remaining 9 pairs are tested as well. There is also a test of unrelated-word pairs. In this test, there are 10 sets of unrelated-word pairs such as "dog-microphone," or "fridge-watch," and the participant usually finds this task much more difficult than the related-word pairs. There are many cases of participants scoring perfectly in the related-word pairs but scoring zero in the unrelated-word pairs. Thus, this test is extremely effective in detecting memory decline. This test is a good way to detect MCI and mild dementia.

2.4 Logical memory

Logical memory is a subtest of the Wechsler Memory Scale-Revised (WMS-R, Wechsler, 1997; the Japanese version translated by Sugishita, 2001). Participants listen to each of two discourses (30 seconds long for each), then are asked to recall the content immediately (immediate recall), and again after a 30 min. delay (delayed recall). The delayed recall is usually much more difficult than the immediate recall. Some participants who obtained the full score in the Mini-Mental State Examination (MMSE) demonstrated extremely low scores in the delayed recall. The test is excellent at detecting mild impairment of recent memory in a few minutes (immediate recall).

2.5 Rey-Osterrieth Complex Figure (Rey complex figure: Meyers & Meyers, 1995)

A complex figure of a 2-D diagram is used in this test. There are several methods for administering this test. In accordance with Yamashita (2007)'s modification, our battery employed coping and drawing it again 30 minutes later from visual memory (delayed recall). Persons with MCI may copy the complex figure, but they show clear difficulty in recalling it 30 minutes later. Further, we can compare the scores with 30 min. delays between the verbal (the logical memory) and visual memory. Some participants who obtain within-age scores in the verbal-related tests mentioned above may demonstrate poor scores in the Rey complex figure task, as this test evaluates visual memory. If the participant has moderate to severe dementia, some of the above tests are often omitted.

2.6 Other types of tests and questionnaires

The cognitive assessment battery of Chiba Rosai Hospital includes several subtests of the Standard Language Test of Aphasia (SLTA) (Standard Language Test of Aphasia Production Committee, 1977), such as naming, comprehension of verbal commands, and calculations. Persons with mild dementia obtain almost perfect scores in the naming and verbal commands subtests. In contrast, persons with frontotemporal dementia sometimes reveal disproportionally low scores in naming and comprehension of verbal commands, compared to their preserved scores on the paired-associate learning test and the Rey-Osterrieth Complex Figure.

Pareidolias are visual hallucination of meaningful objects which arise from ambiguous forms in visual scenes. Yokoi, Nishio, Uchiyama et al., (2014) developed a Noise Pareidolia test. In this test, participants are shown one of 40 pages. Thirty-two pages include figures which look like stains on a wall and they are asked if they can see a human face in it. Eight pages include human faces among the "stains." If they respond that there is a face when a page without a face is presented, a score of "pareidolia" (hallucination) is given. The range of normal score is over 37/40. The test is conducted on participants who are suspected to have dementia with Lewy bodies, in which one of the symptoms is optical illusions.

"Quick questionnaire for forgetfulness" (Karasawa, Yasuma, & Udagawa, 2014) is administered to family members to describe the daily memory-related behaviors of the participant. If the participant is able to respond to this questionnaire, the examiner can compare the answers of the participant and the family member.

When the examiner judges it necessary, the Japanese version of the "The General Health Questionnaire; Japanese version" (GHQ, Nakagawa, & Obo, 1985)" is administered to the participant to measure self-perceived depression, anxiety, insomnia, and lack of social activity.

2.7 The validity of the cognitive assessment battery of Chiba Rosai Hospital

The purpose of our cognitive assessment battery was the early detection of MCI and mild dementia. Yasuda & Nakamura (2000b) investigated discourse comprehension of 16 participants with aphasia (mean = 52.1 years old: they were divided into the two groups), 8 age-matched controls (Healthy Middle: mean = 51.1 years old) and 8 younger controls (Healthy Young: mean = 19.1 years old). They listened to single and four news stories serially presented (for about six minutes in total). The average scores of the two healthy control groups for four news stories were 84.1 % (Healthy Young) and 73.5 % (Heathy Middle). It is noteworthy that the Healthy Middle age group demonstrated a significant decline in remembering the news story presented in the last position (Figure 1-2). In contrast, the Healthy Young

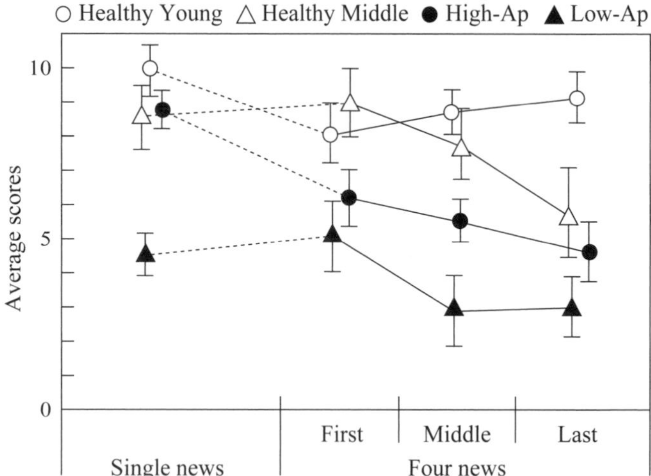

Figure 1-2 Results of listening to four news stories

Notes: Middle = the average score of 2nd and 3rd news. High- and Low-AP: Aphasia groups with high and low scores on the single news.

age group showed a relatively better performance in remembering the last one. A follow-up study was conducted by Bonini & Mansur (2009). The investigation using daily materials such as familiar routes and stories is called as "ecological evaluation" (Hickey, Khayum, & Bourgeois, 2018).

In the subsequent study, Yasuda (2003a) investigated the remembering ability of 3 groups of participants using a 30 min. discourse passage. The participants were 8 persons with mild aphasia (Mild Aphasia mean = 53.6 years old), 7 age-matched controls (Healthy Middle: mean = 49.3 years old), and 10 younger controls (Healthy Young: mean = 19.5 years old). They listened to a 6 min. and a 30 min. discourse passage spoken by a medical practitioner about her therapeutic experiences delivered in a relatively casual manner. The average percentage of the correct scores for the 30 min. passage was 88.3 % in the Healthy Young, 77.3 % in the Healthy Middle. The passages consisted of three stories (first, middle, and last positions), and each position was scored separately. Unexpectedly, lower scores for the last story were not observed for all three groups; the Healthy Young had higher scores for the last story (Figure 1-3).

The 30 min. discourse passage was long but its content was redundant compared to the news story. This may be related to the writing style of the news story, which presented much novel information in a concise fashion.

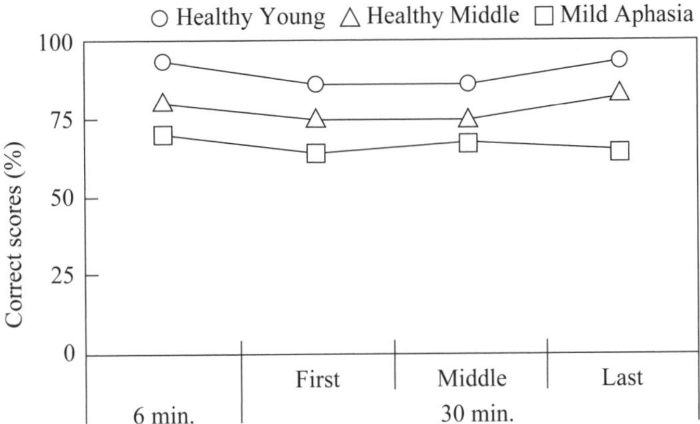

Figure 1-3 Results of listening to 30 min. discourse passages

The observation of age-related reduction of working memory, which was suggested by Salthouse, Mitchell, Skovronek et al. (1989), is complicated by the types of materials used to evaluate working memory performance.

The healthy elderly and persons with MCI sometimes complain about the difficulty in remembering long movies, serialized TV programs, long explanations, etc. Hence, Flores, Bailey, Eisenberg, & Zacks (2017) investigated the long-term recall of movie details one month after viewing the 6 min. movie. It is difficult, however, in clinical settings to evaluate long-term delayed recall. Mahendra (2001) reported that persons with Alzheimer's dementia performed very poorly on the delayed free recall of a short story. Therefore, we decided that the evaluation of immediate recall and 30 min. delayed recall of short stories packed with information was practical. The same may be true for the delayed recall of visual images. However, no such test batteries existed. Consequently, our cognitive assessment battery incorporated the immediate/delay recall of Logical memory from the WMS-R and the copy/delay recall of the Rey complex figure (Yamashita, 2007), in addition to other tests.

Memory impairment is the core symptom of MCI and dementia. Furthermore, as shown in Yasuda & Nakamura (2000b) and Yasuda (2003a), the memory decline may start to occur during the healthy middle age. Healthy people, persons with MCI and dementia are on the same trajectory of chronological memory deterioration. Therefore, in order to detect MCI, we should know the conditions of memory decline for heathy people (see

Section 3.2 in this chapter). A more appropriate memory test battery is expected to be developed in the future.

2.8 Test results and case reports

The results of the cognitive assessment battery are shared with the participants and family members in the Memory Clinic. As shown in Figure 1-4, the battery results are displayed so that participants and family members understand them at a glance. Standard deviations (SD) of age-matched controls for each subtest were obtained from the literature. For each subtest, an adjusted score is calculated using the following equation; $X = 50 - (M - R) \times 10 \div SD$ where M is the mean of age-matched control group, R is the raw score of the participant, SD is the standard deviation and X is the adjusted score. This adjusted score shows where the participant's performance is relative to the distribution of age-matched controls that has 50 as the mean and 10 as the standard deviation.

In the figure, the mean of each subtest of age-matched controls is expressed as the line of 50. The zone of 40 (–1 SD) and below was indicated in gray, suggesting the crucial zone that is to be used as one of the indices for early detection of MCI (Busse, Hensel, Gühne et al., 2006). The SD of the MMSE is not included in the figure since reliable data were not available at that time. A copy of the sheet is given if the participant or his/her family wishes it.

Case No. 1 had a MMSE score of 29, and the scores of other subtests were also above the zone 40 of the age-matched controls (Figure 1-4). He was diagnosed as normal although he complained of forgetfulness (see 5. Clinical history) and minor atrophy was seen on the Voxel-based specific regional analysis for Alzheimer's disease (VSRAD; Sone, Imabayashi, Maikusa et al., 2018). The VSRAD is a software program for measuring the degree of atrophy from the amygdala to the hippocampus by using the Magnetic Resonance Imaging (MRI) image.

Case No. 2 had a MMSE score of 27, and the delayed recall score of the WMS-R was on the borderline. The copy and delayed scores of the Rey complex figure were under –1 SD (i.e., in the grey zone) (Figure 1-5). A SPECT (Single photon emission CT) revealed low blood flow in both of the parietal lobes (Figure 1-6). Consequently, she was diagnosed with possible MCI and advised to be tested again one-year later.

Case No. 3 scored 25 on the MMSE. The scores of memory-related subtests were under –1 SD as shown in the grey zone, excluding the *Kana-*

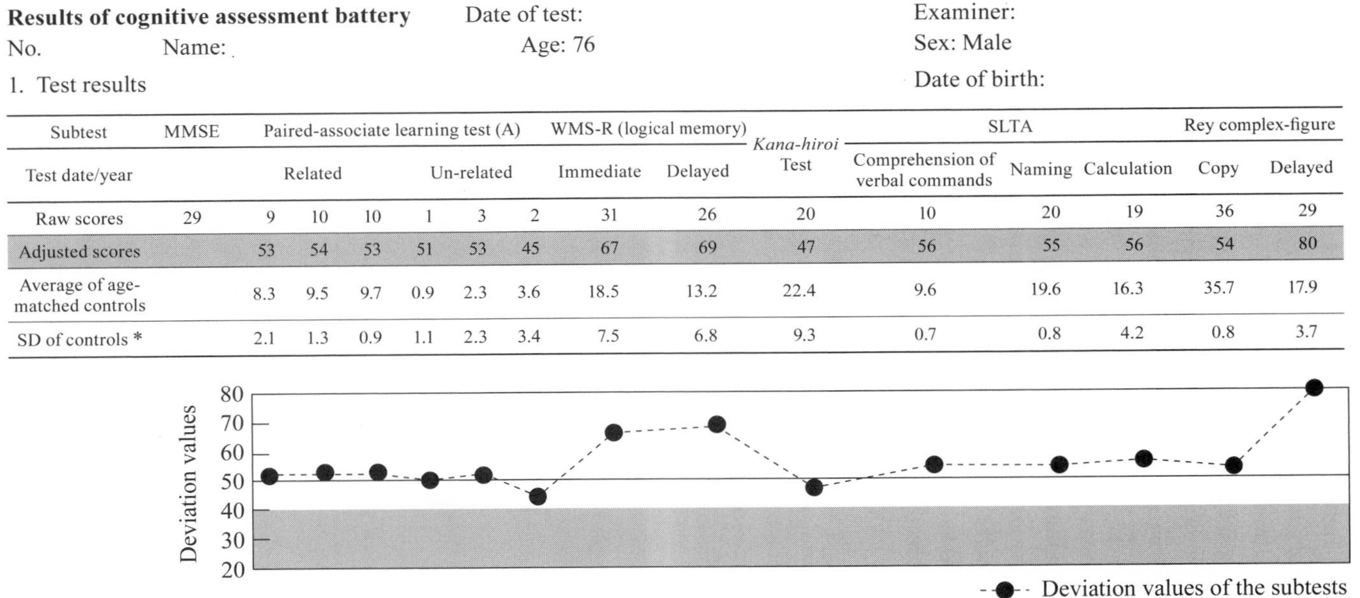

Results of cognitive assessment battery Date of test: Examiner:

No. Name: Age: 76 Sex: Male

1. Test results Date of birth:

Subtest	MMSE	Paired-associate learning test (A)						WMS-R (logical memory)		*Kana-hiroi* Test	SLTA			Rey complex-figure	
Test date/year		Related			Un-related			Immediate	Delayed		Comprehension of verbal commands	Naming	Calculation	Copy	Delayed
Raw scores	29	9	10	10	1	3	2	31	26	20	10	20	19	36	29
Adjusted scores		53	54	53	51	53	45	67	69	47	56	55	56	54	80
Average of age-matched controls		8.3	9.5	9.7	0.9	2.3	3.6	18.5	13.2	22.4	9.6	19.6	16.3	35.7	17.9
SD of controls *		2.1	1.3	0.9	1.1	2.3	3.4	7.5	6.8	9.3	0.7	0.8	4.2	0.8	3.7

Figure 1-4 Results of cognitive assessment battery (Case No. 1)

Note: Standard deviation for 75–79 years old.

2. GHQ 60

Physical symptoms	Anxiety/ insomnia	Social activities	Depressive state
4/7 and over is at moderate clinical stage		3/7 and over is at moderate clinical stage	
/7	/7	/7	/7

3. Quick questionnaire for forgetfulness (Karasawa et al., 2014)

Memory	Language/ behavior	Peripheral symptoms	Total	Pattern
2/10	1/10	0/10	3/30	B: slow progress

☐ Indifference	☐ Anxiety/Insomnia	☐ Persecutory delusion	☐ Change of personality
☐ Hallucination	☐ Clothing	☐ Wondering	☐ Obsessiveness
☐ Day-night reversal	☐ Difficulties in walking		

4. Summary

Dementia *			MCI (based on average SD of memory-related tests)		
Severe	Moderate	Mild	Severe (30–34)	Moderate (35–39)	Mild (40 and over)
			Amnesic single	Amnesic multiple	Others ( )

FAST 2. age-appropriate

Average SD

General	Memory related	Language/calculation	Memory-language/calculation
56	57.1	53.7	3.4

* Degree of dementia by MMSE
☐ 24–30: Normal or MCI
☐ 20–23: Mild dementia
☐ 10–19: Moderate dementia
☐ 0–9: Severe dementia

Figure 1-4 Results of cognitive assessment battery (Case No. 1)

5. Clinical history

According to his family doctor, the client obtained the score of 23 in the Hasegawa Dementia Scale, and he said that he suffered dizziness one year ago. ×× hospital diagnosed that he had no clinical problem. [**Symptoms**] He doesn't remember what his wife talked to him a few days ago. Sometimes, he doesn't remember what he heard earlier in the day. [**Course of the symptoms**] (Information from his family) He cannot find what he is looking for even when it exists in front of him. He gives up his search after a minute and pretends that he doesn't need it after all. He sometimes responds to the conversation in personally convenient ways. He forgets what he has said to his family, and thus he confuses his family members. On November 11, he wanted to go to hospital to be vaccinated against the flu and yet his temperature was as high as 38.6 degrees. But he did not recognize it. Before going to see his doctor, he needed to fill out a form, but his hands were trembling too much to write anything. [**Health history/ clinical history**] At age 66, polyps were found in his large intestine. He currently has no medicines to take. [**Driving**] Everyday [**Smoking**] Smoking (20/a day × 26 years) [Alcohol] Yes. (Japanese *sake*, beer, liqueur, 360 cc/a day × 58 years) [**Currently**] Living with his wife. No problem found in the health check. He joins in a blow-dart circle once a week, and he acts as a caretaker in the club. He plays mahjong every two months. He feels no sign of weakening in his mahjong performance. [**Examiners Impression**] possible MCI

6.

VSRAD *	The degree of atrophy	Area 1 1.30	Area 2 6.22

Cerebral infarction/cerebral hemorrhage/lesion of white matter/ventricular enlargement
Atrophy (hippocampus/parietal lobe/frontal lobe/temporal lobe/occipital lobe)
SPECT: parietal lobe/posterior cingulate gyrus/occipital lobe/temporal lobe/frontal lobe

7.

☐ AD	☐ VaD	☐ MCI
☐ DLB	☐ FTLD	☑ Normal
☐ Alcohol	☐ NPH	☐ Anxiety/insomnia
☐ B1, B12 ↓	☐ Depression	

Figure 1-4 Results of cognitive assessment battery (Case No. 1)
Note: * See Table 8-1 in Chapter 8.

hiroi and the subtests of SLTA. Her SPECT showed low blood flow in the parietal lobe and the posterior cingulate gyrus. She was diagnosed with Alzheimer's disease (Figure 1-7).

Case No. 4 was tested twice, at 72 and 73 years old. At both times, his results were extremely poor in the naming and comprehension of verbal commands subtests, as well as in other memory-related tests. However, the scores for calculations, and copy and delayed tasks of the Rey complex figure remained above the average for age-matched controls. His MRI and SPECT revealed atrophy and low blood flow in the temporal lobe, and he

Results of cognitive assessment battery Date of test: Examiner:

No. Name: Age: 75 Sex: Female

1. Test results Date of birth:

Subtest	MMSE	Paired-associate learning test (A)						WMS-R (logical memory)		*Kana-hiroi* Test	SLTA			Rey complex-figure	
Test date/year		Related			Un-related			Immediate	Delayed		Comprehension of verbal commands	Naming	Calculation	Copy	Delayed
Raw scores	27	10	10	10	0	1	1	11	4	20	10	20	18	34	9
Adjusted scores		58	54	53	42	44	42	40	36	47	56	55	54	29	26
Average of age-matched controls		8.3	9.5	9.7	0.9	2.3	3.6	18.5	13.2	22.4	9.6	19.6	16.3	35.7	17.9
SD of controls *		2.1	1.3	0.9	1.1	2.3	3.4	7.5	6.8	9.3	0.7	0.8	4.2	0.8	3.7

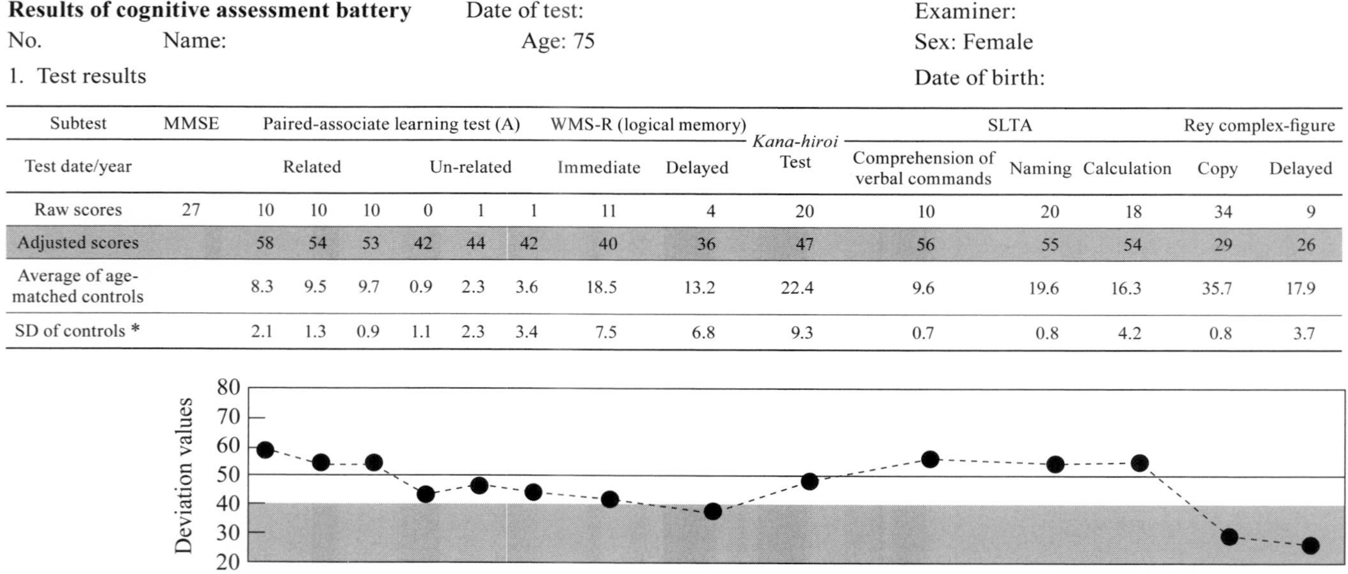

Figure 1-5 Results of cognitive assessment battery (Case No. 2)

Note: Standard deviation for 75–79 years old.

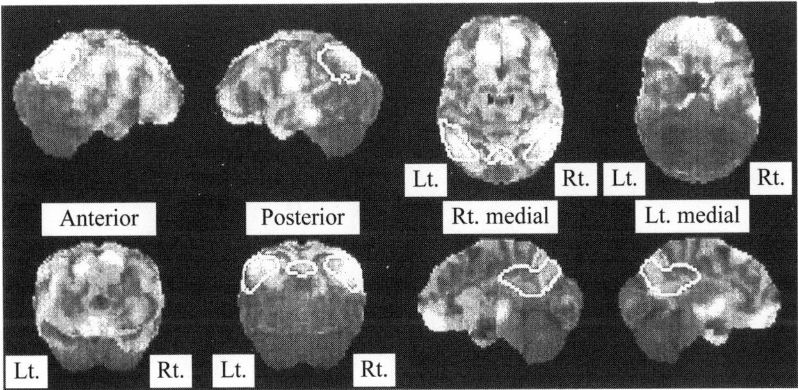

Figure 1-6 Results of SPECT (Case No. 2)

was diagnosed with frontotemporal dementia (Figure 1-8).

2.9 Summary of the cognitive assessment battery

The Japanese Society of Neurology suggests that it is easier to detect MCI if the MMSE and MoCA-J (Montreal Cognitive Assessment-Japanese version) are used together (or, the MMSE and other "complex" memory tests). However, the "delayed recall" of MMSE and MoCA-J were the words recall (3 to 5 words) subtest. As we have seen in the above sections, the "delayed recall" of Logical memory (two short stories) and Rey complex figure are important to detect the MCI. Without executing the Rey complex figure test (copy and delay), we might have overlooked Case No. 2 who was diagnosed as MCI. Therefore, the cognitive assessment battery of Chiba Rosai Hospital includes three kinds of memory tests: paired-associate learning, logical memory, and Rey complex figure (delayed recall). In fact, we experienced that some participants show low scores exclusively in one of the three tests.

As for the detection of mild dementia, the MMSE, or the MMSE combined with the MoCA-J/Word Fluency test are recommended by the Japanese Society of Neurology (2017).

In recent years, a screening test for MCI called "Simple cognitive function scale, *Atamano kenko* [brain health] *check: tee peck*" is available by phone at participants' charge. Two kinds of test for screening dementia are also provided by downloading for free of charge: CADi2 using a tablet (Onoda & Yamaguchi, 2014) and "Moff *Wasurenagusa* [forget-me-not]" (by Moff) using a smartphone. If these tests become available to use at

Results of cognitive assessment battery Date of test: Examiner:

No. Name: Age: 76 Sex: Male

1. Test results Date of birth:

Subtest	MMSE	Paired-associate learning test (A)						WMS-R (logical memory)		*Kana-hiroi* Test	SLTA			Rey complex-figure	
Test date/year		Related			Un-related			Immediate	Delayed		Comprehension of verbal commands	Naming	Calculation	Copy	Delayed
Raw scores	25	4	6	6				4	0	34	10	20	20	34	7
Adjusted scores		29		7	0	0	0	31	31	62	56	55	59	29	21
Average of age-matched controls		8.3	9.5	9.7	0.9	2.3	3.6	18.5	13.2	22.4	9.6	19.6	16.3	35.7	17.9
SD of controls *		2.1	1.3	0.9	1.1	2.3	3.4	7.5	6.8	9.3	0.7	0.8	4.2	0.8	3.7

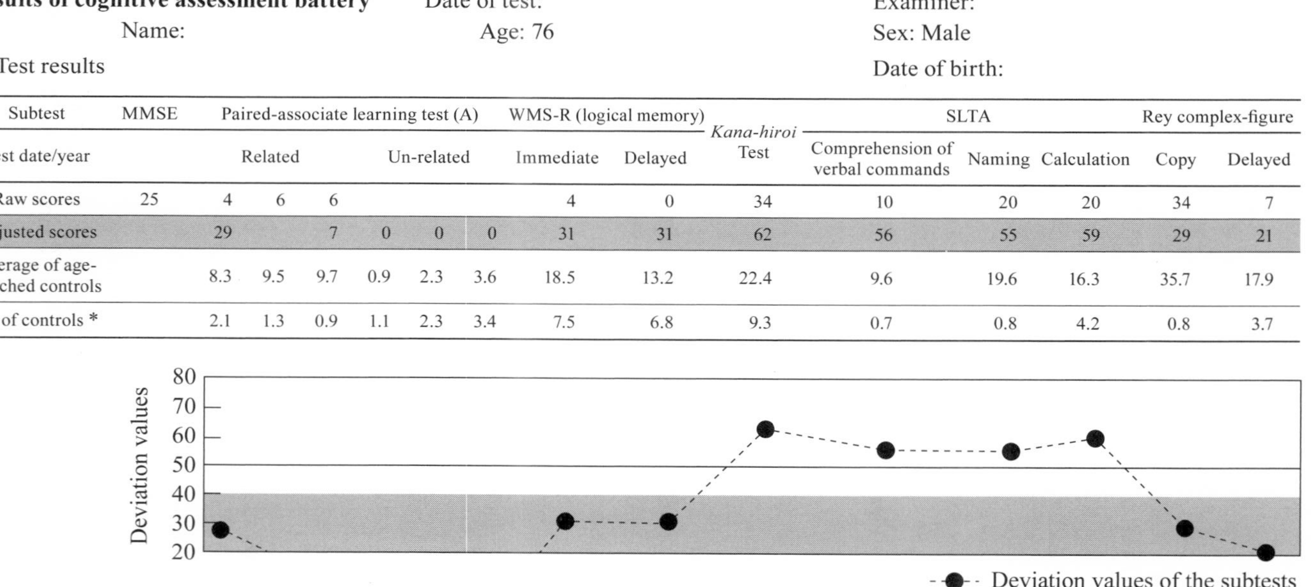

Figure 1-7 Results of cognitive assessment battery (Case No. 3)

Note: Standard deviation for 75–79 years old.

Results of cognitive assessment battery Date of test: February 10 Examiner:

No. Name: Age: 72 Sex: Male

1. Test results Date of birth:

Subtest	MMSE	Paired-associate learning test (A)						WMS-R (logical memory)		*Kana-hiroi* Test	SLTA			Rey complex-figure	
Test date/year		Related			Un-related			Immediate	Delayed		Comprehension of verbal commands	Naming	Calculation	Copy	Delayed
Raw scores	27	3	4	3				4	0	24	(3)	(11)	20	36	28
Adjusted scores		16			0	0	0	31	31	52			59	54	77
Raw scores	27	1	2	1				3	2	19	0	7	20	36	20
Adjusted scores		3			0	0	0	29	34	46			59	54	56
Average of age-matched controls		8.1	9.5	9.8	1.5	3.0	4.7	18.5	13.2	22.4	9.6	19.6	16.3	35.7	17.9
SD of controls *		1.5	0.8	0.6	1.8	2.7	3.3	7.5	6.8	9.3	0.7	0.8	4.2	0.8	3.7

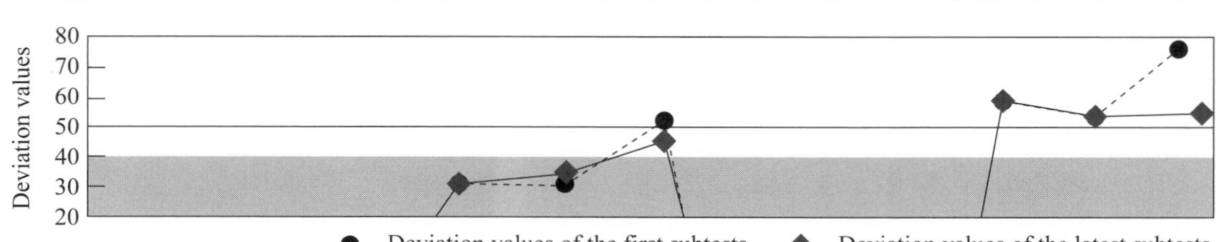

Figure 1-8 Results of cognitive assessment battery (Case No. 4)

Note: Standard deviation for 70–74 years old.

drug stores, convenience stores, and at other public sites, and if the tests are administered periodically, people can monitor their memory abilities over time for maintenance or decline. If their scores were found to be abnormal, they may be automatically advised to go to a doctor with the printed sheets of results.

3. Definitions and clinical stages of MCI and dementia

The diagnostic criteria for dementia in NIA-AA (National Institute of Aging-Alzheimer's Association) is defined as follows: Difficulties in work and daily activities, executive dysfunction, memory impairment, judgement difficulty, disability of visuospatial recognition, language impairment, and behavioral disturbance (McKhann, Knopman, Chertkow et al., 2011). The criteria, however, have been criticized as follows: "The criteria of difficulties in work and daily activities are extremely non-scientific. Although the pathological stage of the brain is the same as other people, the diagnosis may differ depending on the circumstances of the person. For example, some people are required to perform a high level of judgement in an office while others are engaged in domestic life" (Japan Society for Dementia Prevention, 2013). I agree with the ambiguity of this criteria.

The first criteria for a diagnosis of Major Neurocognitive Disorder (dementia) in the Diagnostic and Statistical Manual of Mental Disorders (5th ed.) (DSM-5; American Psychiatric Association, 2013) is "evidence of significant cognitive decline from a previous level of performance in one or more cognitive domains (complex attention, executive function, learning and memory, etc.) As the dementia is defined as progressive, I proposed that the declining ratio of domain (memory) can be used as one of the diagnostic criteria of MCI and dementia (see the section 3.2 MCI below.)

3.1 Types of dementia

Persons with dementia often have responsive behaviors, such as hallucinations, delusions, eating disorders, sleep disorders, irritability, verbal and physical aggressiveness, etc. The pathology causing dementia or dementia-like symptoms are categorized into 13 types. The main types are central nervous degenerative diseases (e.g., Alzheimer's dementia, frontotemporal dementia, and dementia with Lewy bodies, Parkinson's dementia, HIV-related dementia) and vascular dementia (Japanese Society of Neurology, 2017; Hopper, Hickey, & Bourgeois, 2018). The following pathological states are curable by appropriate medical treatments: chronic subdural hematoma, hypothyroidism, vitamin deficiency, high/low blood sugar level, and drug-induced abnormality, etc.

Risk factors for vascular dementia are lack of exercise, obesity, excessive intake of salt, smoking, hyperlipidemia, diabetes, and cardiac disease, which are the same factors as for lifestyle-related diseases. When these risk factors are reduced, vascular dementia can be prevented to some extent. According to Ikota (2016), the number of persons with vascular dementia did not increase in England as the result of a policy to reduce the intake of cigarettes and salt. Therefore, the dementia caused by the central nervous degenerative diseases is truly challenging. Alzheimer's disease is the most prevalent among the diseases. Today, there is no fundamental medical treatment for dementia, although four types of medicines have been approved to delay dementia progressing for several years. In June 2021, the first medicine to cure Alzheimer's disease, ADUHELM (aducanumab) was approved by the FDA (The Food and Drug Administration) of the U.S.A. Regrettably, a lot of questions are raised by many experts about its scientific value.

3.2 MCI (Mild Cognitive Impairment)

MCI is defined as cognitive impairment that persons living with MCI are aware of having memory disturbance. Their memory impairments are also confirmed by memory tests and are recognized by their family/acquaintances, but do not present a major problem in their daily lives. Being able to lead independent daily lives is the critical criterion in distinguishing between MCI and dementia (Ikota, 2016). MCI is characterized by the following symptoms: repetitive utterances, forgetfulness (e.g., leaving a water tap running), being suspicious, quitting hobbies of many years, etc. According to recent reports, persons with MCI show difficulties in using home appliances, in keeping track of finances, and in completing other Instrumental Activities of Daily Living (IADL). Tests for cognitive functions such as the WMS-R's logical memory can detect noticeable decline in persons with MCI. They do not usually have abnormal MRIs but may have abnormal cerebral blood-flow or SPECT scans.

About 5–15 % of persons with MCI are predicted to develop dementia (Japanese Society of Neurology, 2017). On the other hand, Asada (2016) estimated that 50 % of persons with MCI progress into dementia within four years, while approximately 40 % of MCI persons maintain age-related functioning. The difference of the estimated number above might be related to the fact that many people diagnosed with MCI may have other treatable health conditions such as mental disorders, vitamin deficiency, etc. (Arai, 2006).

As for the numerical criteria for the diagnosis of MCI, Petersen, Smith, Waring et al. (1999) suggested that the criterion of their ability measured by memory tests is under -1.5 SD of control average. Meanwhile, the criteria were set by Busse, Hensel, Gühne et al. (2006) under –1 SD, and from –1 SD to –1.5 SD by the NIA-AA (Japanese Society of Neurology, 2017). The cognitive assessment battery by Chiba Rosai Hospital set the grey zone as under –1 SD in order to diagnose a person with possible MCI. I suggest that under –1.25 SD may be the appropriate criterion based on our clinical experience. The validity of these criteria, however, should be examined critically in the future.

In fact, memory ability is largely different among people by nature, and thus it is difficult to set a single criterion. I recommend the following system (Figure 1-9). First, declining ratio of memory ability should be measured for each person annually. If a person's ratio for the past several years is worse than the average of the elderly controls, the person is judged to have a possible MCI. By the traditional simple criteria, the person is judged to have a high-risk of MCI if the test score is lower than the average of the elderly controls. Detecting memory deterioration is, thus, easy for Case 3 in Figure 1-9. But it is relatively difficult for Case 2, and it is significantly hard

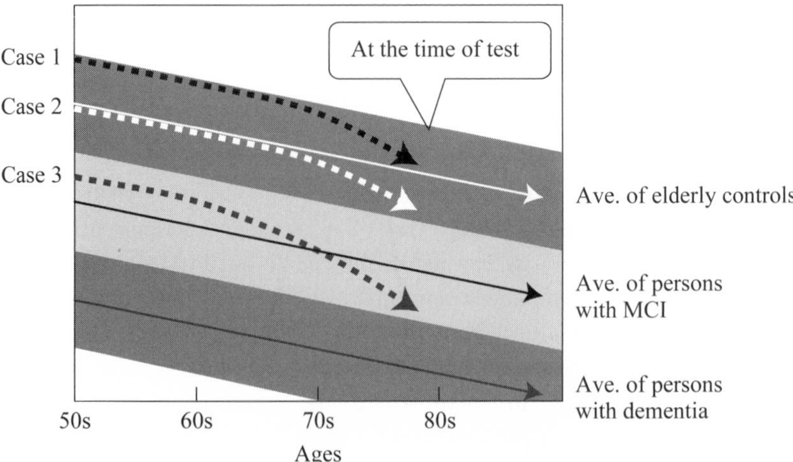

Figure 1-9 Memory deterioration model of three cases

for Case 1. Although Case 1 had a good memory ability previously, his recent memory tests show an abnormal rate of deterioration. Yet his score is still within the average range of controls. According to the simple criteria mentioned above, Case 1 will be at risk of being diagnosed as having no problem. It is ideal to diagnose MCI (and dementia) by the deteriorating ratio of memory ability of an individual person based on data collected regularly. In order to make this decision, we need to find the average ratios of each healthy elderly generation. The delayed recall of discourse may be suitable for the memory test for healthy elderly. We should know the memory deterioration ratios of healthy elderly before discussing the diagnosis of MCI.

4. Evaluation of prevention theories for dementia

Reflecting anxiety about dementia among the healthy elderly, various kinds of prevention theories, brain-activation theories, and so-called "health foods" are eagerly advertised. Even though these theories and foods have reported their effects, it is doubtful whether they have medical evidence. Strict criteria have been applied to recognize "evidence" in the medical academy. For example, a paper submitted to the academy must hold the scientific validity, and it will not be justified until other validated papers report the same results. Recently, the validity of the medicines and treatments are determined by recommendation grades (1: High, and 2: Low) as well as by evidence levels (A: High, B: Medium, C: Low, and D: Very Low). Then, these two categories are combined, for example, 1A is with a high-recommendation and high-evidence or 2C is with a low-recommendation and low-evidence (Japanese Society of Neurology, 2017). It is reasonable to apply these strict criteria for medical validly since they are related to people's health and lives.

"Cochrane Library" on the Internet is assessing from a neutral standpoint not only medicines but also non-pharmacological interventions, supplements, and foods, such as fish oil, ginkgo-leaf extract, Mediterranean diet, and others (Japanese site: http://www.cochrane.org/ja/evidence).

In Japan, there is a book of guidelines called "*Ninchisho shikkan chiryo* [treating dementia] *guideline 2017*" (Japanese Society of Neurology, 2017). It was edited by six Japanese medical academies and shows in the Q&A style the evidence-levels of medicines, related interventions and various products.

The website "Information on safety and effectiveness for heath foods" by the National Institute of Health and Nutrition of Japan is also available (https://hfnet.nibiohn.go.jp/). Reliability is not guaranteed, even if the interventions and products are well known in mass media and popular books. If you have questions about medicines and "health products," it is important to consult with doctors at a memory clinic or hospital.

Related Topics —Warning by the Health and Welfare Ministry of Japan—
A newspaper reported "Dementia is different from forgetfulness of the healthy elderly caused by normal aging." Recently, medicines that allegedly alleviate the forgetfulness of the healthy elderly have been sold on the market. If your forgetfulness is poor enough to cause problems in everyday life, you should see a doctor because you are suspected to have dementia. The Health and Welfare Ministry of Japan requires that pharmaceutical companies should include reminders in the advertisements of their products such as "if dementia is suspected, customers should visit the hospital to receive appropriate medical care." (The *Asahi Shimbun* [newspaper], July 7th, 2017)

4.1 Can supplements prevent dementia?

Today, various supplements are on the market advertising that they prevent the onset of forgetfulness or dementia. The purpose of supplements is to complement deficient substances in the body. For example, iron compounds are used by persons with iron-deficit anemia, and calcium compounds are taken to prevent bone density reduction. Therefore, they have no effect in preventing dementia (Japanese Society of Neurology, 2012). It was also stated by the Japanese Society of Neurology (2017) that "No firm conclusion has been reached that certain foods, nutritive components, or diet patterns would increase or decrease the risk of dementia." At the Memory Clinic, I was told by the wife of a person, whose dementia started in his 50s, that "following a recommendation by a friend of mine (not doctor), I made my husband quit taking medicines prescribed by the Memory Clinic and gave supplements produced by a alleged research institute. But his dementia got worse. So, I resumed giving the medicines for dementia." We should be cautious about advertisements and rumors about the prevention of dementia.

4.2 Can fish and wine prevent dementia?

There are reports that fish and wine, for example, would reduce the onset

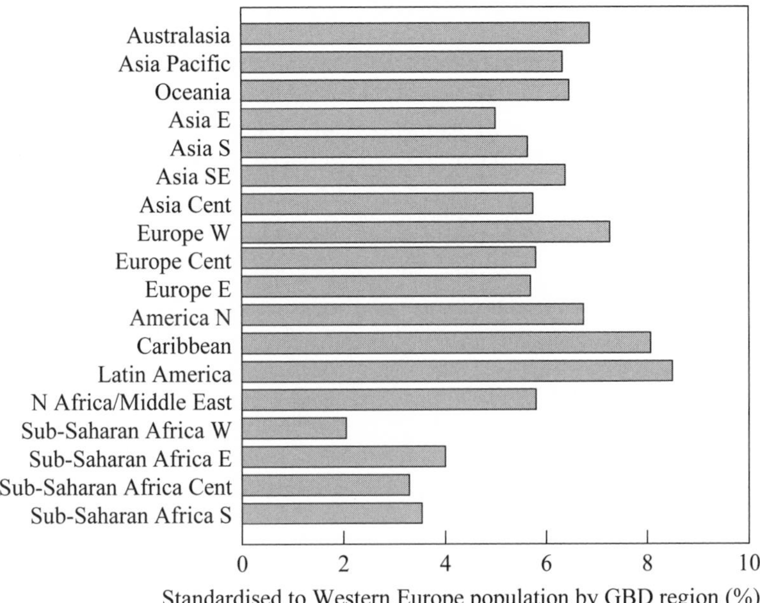

Figure 1-10 Estimated prevalence of dementia for aged 60 and over

Source: Reproduced by the author based on Alzheimer's Disease International (2009). https://www.alz.org/national/documents/report_full_2009worldalzheimerreport.pdf.

risk of dementia. The evidence of these reports, however, ranked as 2C: low-recommendation and low-evidence (Japanese Society of Neurology, 2017). I examined the claim from a different viewpoint. The amount of fish eaten by one person in the U.S.A. on average is one-half of a Japanese person (Japan Fisheries Agency, 2021). The annual amount of wine drunk by one person in the U.S.A. is about one-fifth of a person in Europe (FAOSTAT Food Supply, 2021). If fish and wine, in fact, have effects on the prevention of dementia, the incidence of dementia in the U.S.A. might have been the highest among these counties. However, as shown in Figure 1-10, the prevalence ratio in North America is not much different from that in Europe W (west) and Asia Pacific (Alzheimer's Disease International, 2009). Consequently, the consumption of fish and wine does not seem to contribute to the prevention of dementia in those countries. Even if a difference is found in epidemiological studies between a fish-eating group and a not fish-eating group, the fish-eating effects would be mixed and canceled by other factors when broad areas such as province or countries are compared.

4.3 Can engaging in leisure and mental activities prevent dementia?

Gardening, dancing, cooking and other social activities are often recommended as means to prevent dementia. Reading, *go* (a board game of capturing territory), calculation drills, and other intellectual activities are also suggested that they would prevent cognitive decline among the healthy elderly. However, among clients who came to our Memory Clinic, there were farmers, dance enthusiasts, teachers of mathematics, tax accountants, university teachers, and *go* players with excellent skills. The Japanese Society of Neurology (2017) suggests that "The definition of leisure activities is not clear, and further analyses are needed to reach the conclusion." The evidence level for these activities is reported as low as 2C. Matsuda (2017) indicated that other factors in these activities should be investigated such as a sense of contentment gained from participation, being able to communicate with others, having the time and money to engage in these activities, and having healthy physical and mental conditions that make it possible to do activities.

4.4 Can brain-training prevent dementia?

So-called brain-training such as reading aloud and calculation drills are widely advertised in the media, suggesting that the training can activate the frontal lobe of the brain. Sometimes elderly people are forced to do the brain-training because their family members worry about their risk of developing dementia. In some towns and cities, public taxes are spent to run "dementia prevention classes" in which brain-trainings are offered. Brain images of "activated areas" on MRI in the media lead people to believe that the effects of the training have been proven scientifically. However, as Fujita (2009) explains in his book "*Nou boom no meishin* [superstition about the brain boom]", the brain tends to be temporarily activated by a new stimulus but its activation diminishes as the brain gets used to the new stimulus. Even if the frontal lobe of the brain is activated by the brain-training, it may be useless for Alzheimer's disease because the brain atrophy begins in the parietal lobe, the inner parietal lobe, and the hippocampus, not in the frontal lobe. On the other hand, atrophy or poor blood flow in the frontal lobe are often observed in persons with frontotemporal dementia (FTD). Therefore, so-called brain-training might be more effective for persons with FTD, but evidence of this has not been reported yet.

It is desirable to activate the brain in order to prevent it from "being inactive." However, dementia is a collection of symptoms in which abnormalities occur within nerve cells and the neural networks, and as a result persons with dementia exhibit a variety of cognitive and behavioral impairments, such as memory deficits and difficulty performing daily activities. It is important to show if the "brain-training" would, in fact, improve neuronal physiology (i.e., plaques, tangles, amyloid, Tau), cognition (e.g., memory, visual perception, etc.), and behavioral functioning (e.g., everyday activities). More research is needed.

Alzheimer's disease often begins with an impairment of working memory and episodic memory. An example is forgetting whether he/she has just taken medicines or the date he/she has made an appointment. Therefore, episodic memories should be "activated" if possible. However, recalling daily events is actually difficult for the elderly since their episodic memory has already declined. In contrast, reading aloud and calculation are procedural memory, which tend to be sufficiently sustained among the elderly, even in the persons with mild dementia. When people engage in reading aloud and calculation, they can enjoy a sense of accomplishment, which may make them feel that these tasks are effective or enjoyable. But what the elderly should do is to learn the use of memory aids which will help them overcome the declined episodic memory.

4.5 Can cognitive training prevent dementia?

There are many trials of cognitive training based on computer programs. Owen, Hampshire, Grahn et al. (2010) conducted a study with approximately 10,000 healthy people aged from 18 to 60. The people were divided into three groups according to the types of computer training that they were engaged in. The training types were: 1. Training in logical thinking, planning, and problem solving, 2. Brain-training using a computer, and 3. Training in searching for solutions using websites. The cognitive functions of the participants were evaluated before and after six weeks of training. The results showed that the scores for each task increased in the three groups, but there was no improvement in memory, problem solving, and leaning ability in the tests which were not related to the training tasks. In the literature as well, the effectiveness of cognitive training to prevent MCI from progressing to dementia is not consistent (Japanese Society of Neurology, 2017). Recently, studies are being conducted to find out how cognitive functions are affected by social activities such as engaging in volunteer work, and by new active learning such as using digital devices (see Irazoki, Contreras-Somoza,

Toribio-Guzmán et al. (2020) for other information).

4.6 How to evaluate effectiveness

The scores on the MMSE and other cognitive screening tests are often used to evaluate the effectiveness of interventions. What should be evaluated, however, is whether the frequency of forgetfulness in daily life is really reduced by the intervention. In other words, the evaluation should be aimed at whether the intervention is generalized to functional behaviors in the daily lives of the persons receiving the training. At the Memory Clinic of Chiba Rosai Hospital, persons with MCI/dementia are usually re-tested every 6 months or annually. When the examiner explains that there seems to be no change from the previous test results, the family members would often complain that the persons' memory deterioration is affecting their everyday functioning. This means that cognitive tests do not measure the everyday abilities. Learning effects caused by repeating the tests might also affect the scores of the tests (Yamaguchi, 2010). Yamaguchi (2010) recommended a multidimensional observation scale for the elderly persons (MOSES; Helmes, Csapo, & Short, 1987) and a Japanese version of the Zarit Burden Interview (Arai, Kudo, Hosokawa et al., 1997) which are behavioral-observation scales for everyday activities. As will be described later, observations of specific behaviors that are the targets of the intervention should be evaluated. For example, if a device for automatic voice guidance is used to reduce the frequency of forgetfulness, or for automatic emitted music is used to decrease the frequency of getting angry, the clinician should measure the frequency of forgetfulness and anger episodes before and after the intervention.

Related Topics —Merits and challenges of RCT studies—

Randomized Control Trials (RCTs) are considered to be the experimental method that can achieve the highest level of evidence. In RCT, the effects of a medicine, for instance, are tested between groups of patients taking the real medicine and taking a fake medicine (placebo) without informing the patients which medicine they took. However, RCT studies are difficult to conduct for non-pharmaceutical interventions. For example, RCT cannot be used for evaluating the effects of "real music therapy" and "fake music therapy." Therefore, researchers conduct an RCT where one group gets music therapy and another group gets a different therapy to evaluate relative effects of each (Burgio, Allen-Burge, Roth, Bourgeois et al., 2001).

Another point to consider is that therapeutic effects of non-pharmaceutical interventions are influenced by the individual's interests. (Japanese Society of Neurology, 2017). Since RCT is designed to evaluate effects of a therapy to a certain population, information regarding therapy suitable for an individual with a particular interest is not available in reviews of RTC literature. Such information is likely to be found in case studies or single subject design studies but systematic reviews of such literature are rare. It may well be beneficial to consolidate a summary list of such studies that includes information about characteristics of each participant, therapy tailored to him/her, and response of each participant. Such a list would help clinicians looking for unique and individualized therapy for each participant to obtain information they want, with less time and effort (McDermott, Crellin, Ridder et al., 2012) and Bahar-Fuchs, Clare, & Woods (2013) suggests that non-RCT experiments deserve to get proper evaluations if the experimental procedures are valid.

4.7 Summary of dementia prevention theories

NIH (2019–2020) supports the following approaches: Increasing physical activity, making healthy dietary choices, or getting sufficient sleep may improve cognitive health, as well as computerized cognitive training interventions. The Lancet Commission (Livingston, Sommerlad, Orteta et al., 2017) has similar suggestions. The number of persons with dementia reached 4,620,000 in 2012 in Japan. The number is expected to be 131,500,000 by 2050 in the world and is assumed to increase sharply in developing countries rather than advanced countries. As for MCI, it is estimated to occur in 15–25 % of people aged 65 and over (Japanese Society of Neurology, 2017).

It was discovered recently that nerve cells are newly born in some areas of the brain regardless of age, but the number of cells newly born is a small quantity compared to the size of the brain (Yoneyama, 2010). People lose an average of 5 % of their nerve cells every 10 years after they become 40 years old. Therefore, "The biggest risk for dementia is aging." (Yamaguchi, 2010). Many prevention methods may only have delaying effects for developing dementia (Honma, Yatomi, & Shigeta, 2008), and even those who advocate the prevention of dementia state that "Prevention of dementia does not mean a complete prevention. In fact, it means a delaying of the development of dementia" (Ikota, 2016; Yamaguchi, 2010). In other words, even if we succeed in delaying the development of dementia, the possibility of developing it later on still remains.

Today, anyone can post information on the Internet with or without evidence. It seems that people tend to use the term "prevention of dementia" too easily. I saw that a well-known "brain scientist" said on a TV show: "Chasing flying butterflies will prevent dementia." As a result, many people have come to believe that they can avoid dementia, and some family members are forcing the other members to do drill-training to improve the symptoms of dementia. Many persons with dementia continue driving, and some family members allow them to drive, believing "if they quit driving, they will become more demented." Believing in "prevention theories" could limit the chance to get proper medical treatment. Superficial use of the word "prevention" could also undermine the ideas of creating a "safe society even if we have dementia" proposed by the Alzheimer's Association of Japan (2021). According to Kiyohara (2014), the probability for people over 65 to have dementia by the time they die is 55 %. Recognizing this reality, we should think about what we can do before and after developing dementia.

One of the reasons why "prevention theories" are so popular is because the relationships among memory deterioration by aging, MCI/dementia, and "inactivation of the brain" have been vague and not specified. Figure 1-11 demonstrates the relationships among them (revised from Yasuda (2008b). Memory ability of the healthy elderly is inevitably declining due to aging, although individual differences exist (the healthy declined zone). If a person develops MCI, or dementia, the deterioration of memory ability accelerates further (the MCI/dementia zone). In addition to that, if apathy, depression, loneliness, physical inactivity, etc. are demonstrated and con-

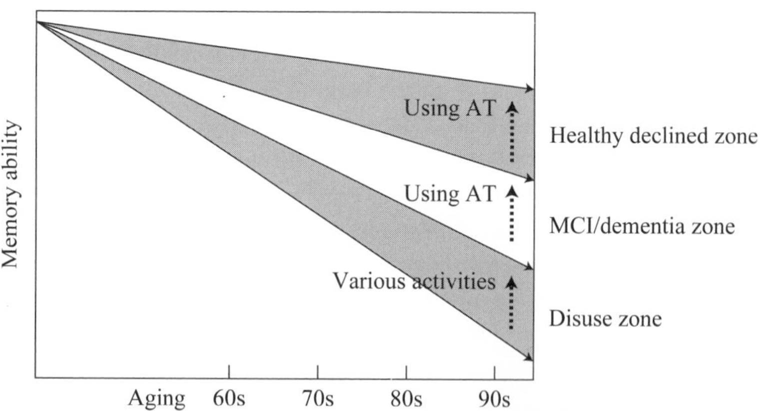

Figure 1-11 Relationships among aging, MCI/dementia, and inactivation

Source: Recreated by the author based on Yasuda (2008b).

tinued over time, memory ability falls into the zone of a "disuse syndrome," or "the inactivity of the brain" (the disuse zone).

In order to prevent people from experiencing the disuse zone, various activities should be encouraged such as conversation, physical exercises, leisure activities, changes in lifestyle, and others. Such activities may raise peoples' scores on memory tests. Recovery, however, stops in the MCI/dementia zone, because the cure for dementia symptoms has not yet been found. Therefore, people have no choice but to employ other approaches for maintaining their memory ability in the healthy declined zone. Yasuda (2007c) and Bourgeois (2014) suggested that memory impairment should be compensated with various Assistive Technology (AT). Utilizing AT may help to raise the impaired memory ability into the healthy declined zone. Even for the healthy elderly, their memory abilities have been declining by aging anyway. Their memory abilities could also be augmented by using ATs such as memo-pads, smartphones, and others.

Related Topics —Programs for the healthy elderly classes—

Drill exercise classes for the healthy elderly have become popular. The first priority, however, should be fall prevention training, because falls cause serious physical and mental effects in the elderly. They should also learn to organize their belongings to be better able to find them, to keep important things together that they need frequently, and to write "ending note" for choosing a surrogate to make decisions for you when they can no longer speak, to decide what medical procedures they would want or not want, and what funeral style they want.

Since episodic memory deteriorates as people get older, it is recommended that they learn how to use various kinds of diaries, a wearable memo-pad (later described), as well as IH (induction heater) cooking heater and other appliances for their safety including surveillance systems for remote family members. They can also learn to use a smartphone or a personal computer as a means to record their daily activities, to remind them of their schedule (alarm feature), to navigate their location (GPS feature), and to communicate by videophone (e.g., Facetime, LINE). Appendices 4 and 5 are the "List of memory strategies for the healthy elderly." By learning and practicing these strategies together with other people, they can raise their information literacy to cope with their declining memory abilities. Another proposal is to build a network by which they can help each other when they develop MCI or dementia (Appendix 2), such as a remote-support network by videophone. Currently, we have started to set up a training system of "Memory Supporter" for promoting AT literacy by the healthy elderly, who give advice to other elders in the community on how to cope with forgetfulness by introducing Low-Tech and Middle-Tech ATs.

5. Rehabilitation for persons with MCI and dementia

“The comprehensive strategy to accelerate dementia measures (New Orange Plan, 2015)” issued by the Health and Welfare Ministry of Japan states that the purposes of rehabilitation for persons with dementia are to evaluate their cognitive and functional abilities, and to encourage them to maintain independent daily lives by maximizing their abilities.

It is commonly accepted that rehabilitation involves four types of approaches: therapeutic, environmental, psychological, and compensatory approaches. Traditionally, most rehabilitation patients have been those with orthopedic impairments, neurological (e.g., stroke), and neurosurgical (e.g., tumor extraction) conditions. Many of them have the potential for natural recovery to a certain extent, except for some patients with degenerative neurological disorders. For the patients whose physical conditions are difficult to overcome, such as limb amputation and chronic hemiplegia, compensatory approaches have been implemented to utilize their remaining abilities.

Rehabilitation for dementia finally started in the 1990s, although the results have been limited due to the effects of memory impairment and the lack of effective medical treatment for continued neurological deterioration. The approaches have been mainly therapeutic, environmental, and psychological approaches. Compensatory approaches for dementia have been slow to be adopted. In fact, there have been relatively few case reports and almost no textbooks written from the standpoint of the compensatory approaches, except for Bourgeois (2014). In addition, there had been few assistive tools developed, which further delayed the adoption of compensatory approaches. Recently, “Flip the Rehab Model” was proposed to promote person-centered care. For this model, the three principles of intervention should be reflected; (1) maximize independent functioning as long as possible; (2) maintain QOL via supported participation and engagement; and (3) emphasize personal relevance and contextual training (Hickey, Khayum, & Bourgeois, 2018). The following is an overview of the rehabilitation roles of physical therapists, occupational therapists, and speech-language pathologists for persons with MCI and dementia.

5.1 Physical therapist

The role of the physical therapist is to maintain ambulation and other physical movements necessary in daily life. Improvements in mobility have been shown to have positive effects on executive and cognitive functions, sleep and bowel movements, quality of life (QOL), social motivation, anxiety, and depression. Physical exercises also have the potential of protective effects against obesity, diabetes, and high blood pressure, and these effects may result in reducing the chances of developing vascular dementia (Ikota, 2016). Responsibilities of the physical therapist are to prevent patients from becoming confined to their beds and falling, while preventing them from a disuse syndrome. For these purposes, therapists provide trainings for the maintenance and improvement of muscular and balance functions, while utilizing compensatory aids such as prosthetic limbs and customized shoes if necessary (Japanese Society of Neurology, 2017).

Persons with dementia tend to lack awareness about their problems, and thus it is important to use cues to alert them to an activity. For example, exercise therapy is found to be enhanced with music. Furthermore, I adopted a strategy in which music was automatically played by an IC recorder at the beginning of walking time to stimulate their motivation. As a result, they walked more with the music than without it. A pedometer on a wristband or wrist-watch style pedometer can be used to monitor the number of steps walked. Some smartphone applications talk to persons and encourage them to do exercises. To keep track of their activity, a memory clinic could loan a pedometer to outpatients and provide a form on which to record how many steps they walked a day.

Recently, simultaneous and multitask training, such as a combination of physical exercise and cognitive tasks (e.g., calculation) are becoming popular among the healthy elderly (Barnes, Santos-Modesitt, Poelke et al., 2013). Because I have observed that many outpatients of the Memory Clinic have had fractures, I have proposed "squatting while reading a newspaper (https://www.youtube.com/watch?v=u_MW0ai2oPI)" and "lifting a leg in four directions during teeth-brushing (https://www.youtube.com/watch?v=oJGDfyavReY)." The latter is aimed to increase muscle strength and balance. The merit of these exercises is that they can become part of the daily routine, just like reading a newspaper and brushing teeth, and they are done usually more than once every day.

5.2 Occupational therapist

Occupational therapists intervene in improving persons' daily lives, work productivity, and the quality of leisure time by having them practice various activities. Occupational activities are expected to preserve the health of the body and mind, as well as motivation and engagement. First, therapists assess the daily needs of patients. Then, they develop goals for each patient based on his/her personality, lifestyle, life history, and cognitive and physical abilities. Occupational therapists also assess the Instrumental Activities of Daily Living (IADLs) of the patient. Persons with dementia have a high risk of falling, getting burned, causing a fire, and being involved in other domestic accidents. Therapists often provide environmental modification and home health aides.

For persons with severe dementia, therapists identify meaningful tasks that they can still enjoy because of preserved procedural memory, such as knitting, cutting vegetables, playing the piano and others. Advanced Activities of Daily Living (AADL) are QOL-related activities such as communicating with friends, enjoying hobbies, and participating in social activities. Maintaining AADL activities often start to become difficult when a person develops MCI. Therapists, therefore, should offer appropriate and timely support to persons at that stage, and as their cognitive abilities deteriorate.

5.3 Speech-language pathologist

Speech-language pathologists (SLP) assess persons with aphasia, apraxia, agnosia, and other brain dysfunctions such as MCI, dementia, and brain injuries. They assess cognitive functions, such as expressive and receptive language, memory, executive functioning, and visual perception. SLPs also provide training for communication, memory, and other cognitive functions, as well as swallowing difficulties.

SLPs performs cognitive interventions for persons with memory impairments and dementia. According to Hickey & Bourgeois (2018), cognitive interventions are classified into three types: cognitive stimulation, cognitive training, and cognitive rehabilitation. Cognitive stimulation is an intervention approach that is often performed in groups, and involves engaging the individual in stimulating activities and discussions (e.g., reminiscence therapy, reality orientation, and social activity, etc.).

Cognitive training uses structured interventions with specific exercise or tasks (e.g., attention, execute functions, episodic memory). This type of treatment is usually executed individually, and may often be done on computers. Participants tend to improve only on the trained tasks or tests with similar tasks. Improvements in overall cognitive functioning or generalization to other tasks should not be expected from cognitive training tasks.

Cognitive rehabilitation is the most person-centered and ecologically valid of the three types of cognitive interventions. The purpose of cognitive rehabilitation is to maximize independence and meaningful engagement in daily life using individualized strategies that capitalize on preserved strengths. Treatment strategies used in cognitive rehabilitation for memory deficits have been described as either internal or external in focus. Internal strategies require conscious rehearsal, and the ability to apply them at the relevant time. External strategies, or external cueing systems and aids compensate for memory and communication deficits by capitalizing on preserved strengths.

As for training procedures, evidence is accumulating that persons with mild to moderate dementia can learn new information, or relearn "forgotten" information, using appropriate training strategies, such as spaced retrieval training, errorless learning, vanishing cues, etc. Training can ensure that external memory aids are used routinely. Successful cognitive rehabilitation, particularly using spaced retrieval training and eternal memory aids, has been reported in the literature. Persons with mild to moderate dementia can learn or relearn information or skills, and they can use external memory aids to compensate for their deficits. See Hickey & Bourgeois (2018) for details.

Recently, in hospitals and care facilities for the elderly, a short-term intensive rehabilitation course has been implemented in Japan, but the contents of rehabilitation for dementia are in many cases cognitive training and calculation worksheets. Training to use ATs should be included considering the person's daily life after discharge. Bourgeois (2014) suggests that compensatory approaches are better than training of memory for persons with dementia because their memory has already deteriorated, and it will degenerate further. For example, training to look at a calendar is much better for them rather than training to memorize the day. I agree with her suggestion that the methods acquired by compensatory approaches would well be generalized to their daily lives. Hereafter, SLPs should implement compensatory approaches and utilize various types of ATs for assisting persons in their daily lives.

6. Daily support by using Assistive Technology

At present, clinicians explain the symptoms of dementia to persons, and instruct the family members to take reflective attitudes when the person exhibits responsive behaviors. Furthermore, redirection techniques are recommended in which the responsive behaviors should be redirected to more desirable activities. In this approach, the following is proposed to the family member: "When a person tries to go outdoors alone, gently suggest an alternate activity; for example, "Let's go pick some flowers in the garden and then put them in a vase." This is certainly one of the basic approaches for caring for persons with dementia, and some family members may be able to do this. In reality, however, they may need training and support in the home to implement suggested strategies successfully.

They may experience many stressors that make caregiving difficult. For example, if a family member has to quit his/her job in order to take care of the person with dementia, he/she will lose financial resources. When persons' responsive behaviors increase in frequency and severity, there are reports of abuse or nursing home placement. Professionals in this field must identify a variety of resources to address and reduce family members' burdens. One possibility is the compensatory approach of using AT, which aims to reduce the family members' burden and support the daily lives of persons with MCI and dementia.

6.1 MCI and dementia persons have "information impairment"

The main impairment of MCI and dementia is memory impairment (Yasuda, 2007c). Memory impairment is considered to be the synonym of "**information impairment**" by which persons are unable to retrieve information when needed. Even if the information is stored in long-term memory, it is difficult to retrieve and utilize. For example, some persons are unable to remember the location of the toilet, leading to incontinence. Some persons try to go to work because they cannot remember that they have retired. They forget where they put their wallet just a minute ago, leading to delusions of theft. They mistake someone else as their wife because they cannot recognize their aging wife's face.

Since information impairment produces the above symptoms, a way to support memory is to provide the needed information in a meaningful way. For example, when a person with dementia approaches the bathroom, an AT can tell him/her the toilet is nearby. When they go to the door to leave for work, an AT can tell him/her "you have already retired," or "It's time to wash the dishes in the kitchen." Some forms of AT, like a memory book or a reminder card can provide persons with desired information before they ask questions repeatedly. Or AT in the form of two photographs can show the wife's photo at a younger age and her current age in order to facilitate recognition of the current face of the wife. Clinicians need to learn about various ATs and how to implement them for specific behaviors.

To maximize the effectiveness of the compensatory AT approach, family members and persons with dementia have to have this information before the problems become overwhelming. I call this "**the strategy of providing information in advance**." Some persons may not accept when they are given correct information. In such a case, family members are allowed to present information that is not true but the person can accept. For example, when they say, "This is not my home, so I am leaving now," do not reply "This is your current home." Instead, family members could say, "You are visiting your daughter's home, so stay here tonight." It may be necessary to repeat this information as many times as the person requires. A helpful AT approach would be to use a memo-pad, an IC recorder, smartphone, and other kinds of AT to present the information the person with dementia needs. Information to be presented by ATs could also include music, moving images, and others.

6.2 History of humans and information

Personal computers do not necessarily store all the memory in the hardware, but in an external memory medium such as USB, SD card, etc. Historically, written language systems, including alphabets and other kinds of characters and letters, were a kind of compensatory and external means of human memory. Writing was developed for recording a tribe's history; and they wrote on stones, glass, or on paper, rather than depending on the brain to remember. In fact, there used to be people who specialized in memorizing in the age before the written word, and they memorized the history of their tribe (the oral history approach). Presently everyone uses AT in some form, even healthy people and children who use calendars, planners, smartphones, and other note-taking systems. Thus, persons with memory impairment would already know how to use AT because they used it throughout their life. They may just need to be reminded to use their external memory media. The elderly sometimes say that keeping a diary makes their memory deteriorate because they are not using their brain to remember. But such a claim is questionable for people whose memory has already been deteriorating. After all, memory deterioration will continue as they get older. Therefore, they should be encouraged to use AT for information storage and retrieval as soon as possible.

6.3 Application of AT

Many kinds of prostheses and tools have been used in physical therapy and occupational therapy such as canes, wheelchairs, artificial limbs, etc. for daily activities. Glasses and hearing aids are also recommended for people with poor eyesight and hearing (Bourgeois, 2014). In the same way, AT should be suggested for persons with MCI and dementia. An AT, for example, could help them remember to take their medicines. Their family members should also be provided with ATs, which may ease the burden of dealing with repetitive questions. In order to maintain a good quality of life, the utilization of remaining abilities and the use of ATs are the core of rehabilitation for persons with MCI and dementia. It is also ideal for the healthy elderly to learn in advance how to use ATs. If they learn and start using ATs for their impending memory decline, the knowledge and practice will reduce their problems even if they develop MCI or dementia (Appendices 4 and 5).

6.4 Effectiveness of AT

Greenaway, Duncan, & Smith (2013) suggested that keeping schedules in calendars and notebooks by persons with MCI will be effective in maintaining ADLs, in building a sense of achievement, and in reducing the burden on family members. However, there have been few reports of ATs for persons with MCI and dementia. Further, the ATs reported so far were traditional ATs and practices such as keeping household accounts, keeping a diary, making a note, writing a daily schedule on a whiteboard, remembering one's life by looking at photo albums, sticking labels on shelves, and hanging a simple sign on the door of the toilet (Honma et al., 2008). It is obvious that the range of problems to be resolved by these traditional ATs is narrow and their users may be limited to persons with MCI or mild dementia.

About 10 years ago, incidents of forgetting to turn off the gas, burning a cooking pot and overflowing bathtub water were often reported at memory clinics. Recently, such incidents are hardly heard of because of the use of a sensor for preventing people from cooking a pot without liquid in it and a device to stop the water supply automatically. These devices have served the role of AT, by preventing the incidents caused by memory impairments. Today we are blessed with having a wider variety of ATs. For example, we can find lost people, or lost belongings, by using GPS and Bluetooth devices, and we can trace their movement by using a smartphone. High resolution cameras are now available at low prices to be used to observe behaviors all day. In 2017, the *Lancet* added "Technology" for the first time to one of the ten important messages for supporting persons with dementia and argued that AT should be used in the diagnosis of dementia, in daily observation, and in supporting family members (Livingston et al., 2017). Japanese Society of Neurology (2017) recommended also for the first time to utilize Information Technology (IT) devices for training and daily supports such as IT-using calendars and notebooks, though their evidence level is still as low as 2C. The situation seems to be much better now compared with the time when my colleagues and I recommended the use of IT in 2003. At that time, a glacial stare was given to us by the leaders of dementia-related academic and family members' societies.

6.5 For further development of AT

Many staff members in the caring professions who have had limited experiences of implementing ATs would say that electronic devices seem to lack friendliness for the elderly. I have, however, received the following reaction from a person with MCI. He was waiting in front of the IC Recorder to "greet" my voice that comes out automatically every morning. Later, the person told me that "I was very happy to hear the voice of a person who is not a family member. I thank you for concerning yourself about me, even if the voice was a recorded one." Today, you can talk anytime with your family members or friends by using a videophone. Whether you talk in a live situation or online is simply a matter of communication means. If these means are used to increase the opportunities of conversation, it would lessen, for instance, loneliness. It will be very helpful to search for other possible ATs at stores and on the Internet, while you create and apply new ATs to improve the QOL of persons with dementia.

People will not lose all of their abilities when they develop MCI and dementia. With the use of their remaining abilities and appropriate AT, they might be able to continue their jobs. Persons with moderate stage dementia may continue living independently, and persons in the severe stage may be given ways to enjoy life and to communicate with others. However, the speed of deterioration and the range of cognitive impairments differ among persons, requiring different intervention methods. Ideally, hundreds of kinds of ATs should be created for hundreds of different disabilities. Therefore, professionals should make an effort to familiarize themselves with a wide range of ATs in advance, as well as their application methods, for the variety of persons they will encounter.

Sometimes people want to know if using ATs can prevent persons with dementia from getting worse. AT has compensatory and augmentative roles for supporting their abilities, and AT may increase their QOL. The progression of dementia cannot be prevented at this time. Even using AT cannot stop the progression. These approaches, therefore, are irrelevant to the prevention of disease. Many persons with dementia found it difficult to control home-electronic appliances as their cognitive functions deteriorated. When dementia is progressing, the AT may need to be modified so that the person's remaining abilities are utilized to the maximum at each stage.

Although the nuclearization of families has been increasing, the Japanese government has been decreasing the service components covered by the Long-Term Care Insurance. In these situations, more stresses are being placed upon the family members and demands for the usage of AT will inevitably increase. It is urgent that more efficient AT should be developed by studying and working, not only with persons with dementia, family members, and experts in this field, but also with engineers, designers, and psychologists, etc.

Many of the experiments described in this book were not evaluated using RCT (Randomized Controlled Trials). As a result, their evidence level is low. However, the case studies documenting behavioral changes before and after the intervention by AT are promising. It has been the aim of this book to provide various ideas for future studies. I have not applied for patents for the various ATs or designs that I have developed and introduced here, except for some goods available commercially. It is expected that the younger professionals in the field will freely modify and apply the ATs introduced here. As a result, the effects, as well as the limitation of these ATs, will clearly be revealed. Based on these experiences, I hope that new and more effective ATs along with their application methods will be developed.

CHAPTER TWO

Daily support using Low-Tech AT

There are ATs that are specifically designed to assist memory, some of which can be operated by hand and require no electricity, and are called Low-Tech AT in this book. The advantage of Low-Tech ATs is that they can be used intuitively (Hickey & Bourgeois, 2018). Ideal ATs should be usable without much training and/or reading manuals, and easy to maintain. In this chapter, special diaries are introduced, followed by wearable memo pads, calendars, and message boards. These ATs are designed for persons with memory impairments such as healthy elderly with forgetfulness, and persons with MCI and dementia, cerebral infarction/hemorrhage, or brain dysfunctions caused by head injuries. Most of the Low-Tech ATs introduced have been developed by me, since there had been few such ATs. Recently, even healthy-middle-aged people seem to become forgetful due to information overload in modern society. In the last section of this chapter, I propose a newly developed diary for the healthy-middle-aged/elderly and explain how to use it so that writing and viewing the diary becomes easy.

1. New Memory Support Diary

Writing up documents and keeping them is an important practice in accounting as well as in other jobs. Accurate and detailed records should also be required for supporting the daily lives of persons with memory impairment. The primary method for managing memory impairment is to keep a diary and to use the diary to recall information when needed. It is common for professionals to give instructions to the persons to "keep a diary" or "take notes." This instruction, however, is not often helpful because diaries avail-

Date:	Weather:	What's important today

Today's plan	Done	What I did and who I met

Financial records		Meals and menu		Medication and time	Notes
		Breakfast			
		Lunch			
		Dinner			
		Snack			

Schedule (write until that day)	Things to remember (write until you memorize)	Health
Month Date Day Time		Blood pressure: Pulse:
Month Date Day Time		Weight: Temperature:
Month Date Day Time		Blood sugar: Constipation:
Month Date Day Time		Number of steps: Walking time:
		Wake-up time: Bedtime:

Place to put	Wallet	Glasses	Phone	Bag	Watch	Key ( )	Key ( )	
Confirmation								

Figure 2-1 The New Memory Support Diary
Source: Recreated by the author based on Yasuda (2013a).

able on the market are designed for healthy normal people and there have been no suitable diaries for the memory impaired. Specifically, there does not seem to have been any discussion about what the appropriate format of a diary would be for the memory impaired person, except by Sohlberg & Mateer (1989). After much consideration I published a special diary for memory impaired people in 2007. The revised edition was published in 2013 (Yasuda, 2013a) as "*Shin Kioku Sapoto Cho* [New Memory Support Diary] (https://escor.co.jp/products_list/products_list05.html) (Figure 2-1).

The New Memory Support Diary has a particular format that is different from existing diaries (Table 2-1). A double-page spread is set up for keeping a log for one day. The left page is blank. The right page is divided into several sections to fill in; categories are meals, health, schedule, and belongings the user tends to misplace. Writing into these sections helps the users to find what information they might need later. The size of each section fits that of common sticky-notes (e.g., Post-it® in 5 × 7.5 cm size) available on the market (see Table 2-1 for details of each section). Users are advised to bring sticky-notes with them when they go out and write memos on them. The sticky-notes, then, should be placed in their New Memory Support Diary after they come home. In this way, the sticky-notes can become part of the daily log in the diary. This will prevent the loss of their sticky-notes and their important information. The same is true for scratch memo paper.

1.1 How to use the New Memory Support Diary

People usually say they will write in the diary when I recommend them to do so but many find it difficult due to their prospective memory impairment. Thus, it is recommended that a user and his/her family members make it an everyday routine to write and review the diary at a certain time of the day. The use of a smartphone or an IC recorder to remind the user with an alarm or a voice instruction is also recommended (see Chapter 3 for more information).

If the diary is put away in a desk, users are apt to forget to write in the diary. The New Memory Support Diary has a hole which can be used to tie it up to somewhere with a string, and users can also attach a pen with a string to the diary. This can prevent them from losing the diary and pens. The diary can be placed on the refrigerator door with a magnetic clip, and in this case, users can fill in the diary while standing.

When a user who has kept a dairy for years begins to feel that keeping

Table 2-1 Contents of each section in the New Memory Support Diary

Today's plan: Fill in "today's plan" in the morning or on the previous day, for example, "go to hospital at 9"or "weeding the garden." When the task is completed, check the item and write down the time. Family members could write messages in the diary, such as "Please cook curry for dinner". Thus, it might be a good idea for the user and his/her family members to share the diary. For example, a user would write on the right page, and a family member would write his/her schedule on the left page so that they can recognize each other's schedule.
Meals: Writing down what a user ate is for monitoring healthy eating practices and to prevent unhealthy food choices such as eating the same food day after day. It is desirable to write down immediately after the meal, or before the meal.
Financial records: Monitoring income and expenses is one of the means to prevent users from having the delusion that their money is being stolen. Receipts can be glued on the left blank page, and total amount spent can be written in this section on the right page.
Things to remember: In order to reduce the frequency of questions being asked repeatedly (e.g., "Where is my bankbook?"), write in what a user should remember. Family members should suggest the user to look up the section of diary whenever s/he asks the same questions. This will avoid the vicious circle of repeating the same questions and answers that leaves both parties frustrated. Writing is also helpful for the user to remember the whereabouts of important items (e.g., "My glasses are near the entrance door.") and to form necessary habits (e.g., "I need to take a memo pad when I go shopping.").
Health: The following health conditions and exercises may be written; weight, blood pressure, bowel movements, the number of steps walked, as recommended by the physician to monitor health conditions and healthy behaviors.
Medication: Write down the names of medicines, and when they should be taken. It is helpful to fill in the section so that they can check off when they took their medicines. This is especially important when a user has conditions such as diabetes.
Schedule: Even if the schedule is written on a calendar, people often forget to look at the calendar. Thus, users are encouraged to write down their plans every day until the plans are executed. It may be a good idea that they write in a plan while counting down its date, such as "5 days until the trip" or "2 days left in the trip." If a user has moderate dementia, his/her family member can review the diary with him/her on a daily basis and discuss what's coming up in the near future.
The blank page: The left-side page of the double-page spread is a blank page. Users could glue shopping receipts, directions for medicines, photos, newspaper clippings, and so forth, which will help the users recall the information later. A shopping list (sticky-note) can be attached to the diary and users can take the list with them when going shopping. However, some users tend to buy the same things repeatedly which are not on the shopping list. In this case, users may also write down what they should not buy. The users could also write down what they heard in conversations such as a person's name and messages that they want to remember. The page is also used for on-paper calculations, and/or drawing what the users saw. Usually, users throw away sticky-notes or scratch memo papers after they finish the tasks written on them. However, I recommend the users to check off "finished" tasks on the notes but glue the notes on the left page because these notes can be used to remind the users of what they have done that day.

a diary is laborious, his/her clinician should investigate how he/she deals with the diary. Some people may become frustrated about not remembering things to write if they routinely write the diary at night. In such a case, the clinician may suggest the user to keep the diary open on the desk all day so that he/she can write in it whenever he/she wants. Alternatively, the clinician may suggest the user to routinely write in the diary multiple times a day (e.g., after each meal).

Commentators in the media would often say that "In order to strengthen memory ability, recalling and writing what happened two days ago in the diary is recommended." However, this claim is impractical because the elderly who forget about events from this morning or yesterday cannot write about what happened two days ago. A more practical way to train memory is writing in a diary on the day, and after several days recall the contents and check it against what they wrote. Some people argue that if they keep a diary, they will stop making efforts to remember what happened in the day. Whether or not, many of us cannot recall what we ate three days ago without writing it down in the diary. Some people stop keeping a diary saying they have nothing to write because nothing new happens every day. In this case, they should vary their daily lives to flee from the state of "inactivity." Or I recommend that they write current events from newspapers, and what they saw on TV in addition to personal events.

In activity classes for the elderly, members may have opportunities to show their diaries to other members and to talk about recent events looking at their own diary. This will motivate other members to write something in their diary as well as to support their episodic memory. There are some users who kept the New Memory Support Diary for ten years. There is also a person with MCI who said, "As I live alone, I cannot live without relying on this diary which I wrote." It may take several months before persons get used to keeping the diary. Accordingly, as soon as people start being unable to recall the events of the day, they should begin to keep a diary, or change a habit of writing it at night to writing in it whenever things happen.

2. Wearable memo-pads

I recommended that persons with memory impairments write in a diary throughout the day. However, it may not be easy for them to do if the diary is not placed in the same location every day. They may forget what they were going to write before they find it. Alternatively, if people carry a memo-pad with them, they can write on it every time they have something they want to remember. But this is not as easy as it sounds. In the first place, they may forget to carry the pad. Persons with moderate, or severe memory impairment may forget that they are carrying the pad with them. At the Memory Clinic I sometimes saw men take a memo-pad out of their pockets to write on, but there were few women doing so because women's clothing often has no pockets. Women usually carry a bag, but they may forget to take a memo-pad out of the bag if it is not visible, or it may seem troublesome to take it out.

An ideal solution is to use a memo-pad that is wearable on their clothes, or body. This type of pad allows them to make notes immediately after they decide to write something, without the trouble of taking it out of a pocket or bag. However, no such memo-pads have been described in the literature, except some for persons with severe dementia (Bourgeois, 2014). I, therefore, developed various kinds of wearable memo-pads that will be described in this chapter. On the English version of my website (https://gensoshi.jimdofree.com/home-pages-for-english/ or, search with "Kiyoshi Yasuda homepage), the directions for how to make some of them are shown.

2.1 Sticky-note type

Sticking a written memo on the back of the hand is very helpful for a quick and easy reminder. Recently, unique sticky-notes are available on which the entire back has glue (Figure 2-2). The adhesive is so strong that the sticky-notes do not drop off for several hours even from hands or the sleeves of clothing. If you put several layers of sticky-notes on your arm, you do not need to stick a new one again after you write a memo. Important messages

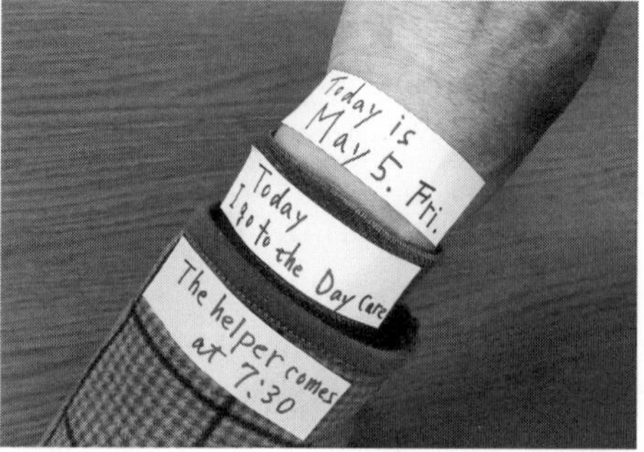

Figure 2-2 Sticky-notes which have glue on entire back

or reminders should be stuck on both arms. The sticky-note can also be placed on the screen or the band of a watch. Recently, sticky-notes that can be copied are on sale. For instance, one can be pasted in a diary and the other can be pasted on an appliance. Flexible band-type memo-pads "WEMO; Wearable Memos" are on sale (https://www.japantrendshop.com/wemo-wearable-memo-p-4422.html). The written memos can be erased with a finger or an eraser. The back side of the ID card holders sold by the same company are made of the same material as above, so you can write and erase memos.

2.2 Bracelet-type with wristwatch

I developed the bracelet-type memo-pad in 1987 initially for persons with communication impairments as a tool of written conversation (Figure 2-3). The sensation of wearing the bracelet on the skin tends to help people remember it is there, or notice if it is not there. This is also useful for persons with memory impairments. They can see the memo-pad easily and can make a note whenever they want. Several blank sheets in clear files are layered under the cover of the bracelet, so that users can use separate sheets for different categories of information, such as telephone numbers and ID numbers, etc. Another layer of sheets for memo taking is also stacked under the bottom cover. Simply lifting the cover allows users to easily find the

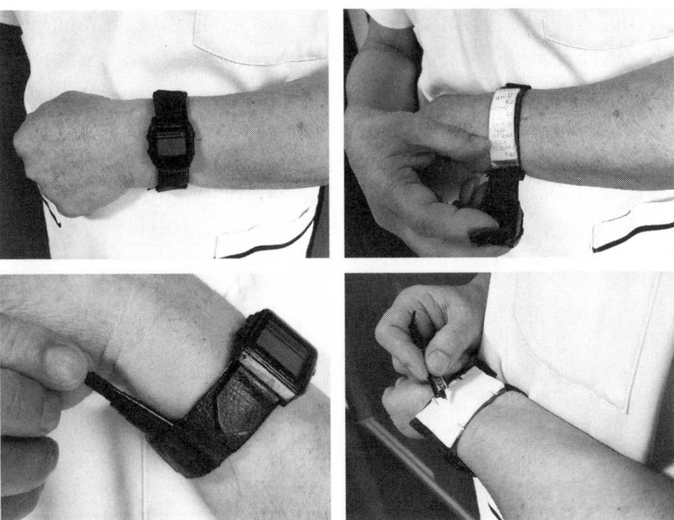

Figure 2-3 Bracelet-type memo-pad with a wristwatch

desired information. I also developed a convenient retractable pen that can be placed into a capsule in the bracelet and is easily retrieved when they need to write a note. The alarm of the wristwatch, if attached on the top cover of bracelet, can be set to alert the user to refer to the memo-pad notes regularly. The design of this pad is on my website for your reference.

2.3 Name-tag type

Name-tags can be modified to include scratch memo paper for writing notes and may be convenient for workers (Figure 2-4). Two name-tags are taped together at their lower edges. At their upper edges, the two name-tags can be attached or detached by two magnets on both the sides (also applied to some of the memo-pads described in this chapter). Scratch paper and a pencil can be inserted in between the two name-tags. Users can look at memos when they open the front tag, for instance to confirm the time of a meeting. There was a woman who inserted a photo of flowers into the front tag and was pleased to wear this name-tag. The "Reversible ID card holder" and "The name card Florist" by Loft are two-ply name cards (https://www.loft.co.jp/). They are easy to modify so as to put scratch memo paper/sticky-note on both the inner sides. Recently, "Pemo ID" which has pens and sticky-notes was released by Zebra.

Persons with memory impairments may forget that they are wearing a memo-pad. An easy way to remind them to read their memos is to attach a string to the upper side of the two cards and let the front tag hang open at 90 degrees. This allows users to notice the card and read it whenever they look down or their arm touches it. Family members can write down the answers to repetitive questions on the memo card and instruct the users to look at the card when asked, thus avoiding the vicious cycle of "ask-reply" (the right-hand photo in Figure 2-4). This "**half-opening system**" can also

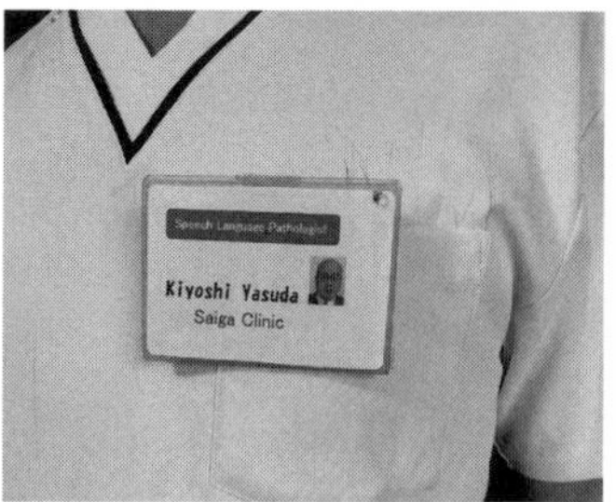

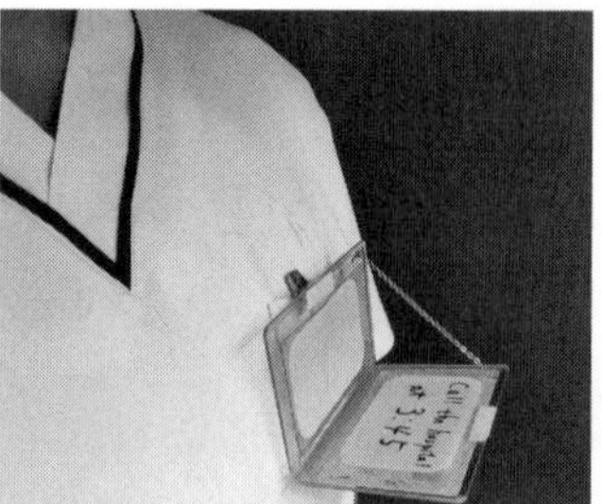

Figure 2-4 Name-tag type memo-pad and half-opening system

be applied to the following memo-pads.

2.4 Waist-type

The above name-tag type of memo-pad or commercially available business card cases can be modified into the waist-type memo-pads by inserting sticky-notes, scratch memo paper, and pens (Figure 2-5). Then attach a clip on the back of the name-tag/case, with which the name-tag/case can be hung on the belt, or on the edge of the pants. Adding a retractable or expandable cord between the clip and the name-tag/case can make it easy for users to write on the memo-pad by stretching the cord.

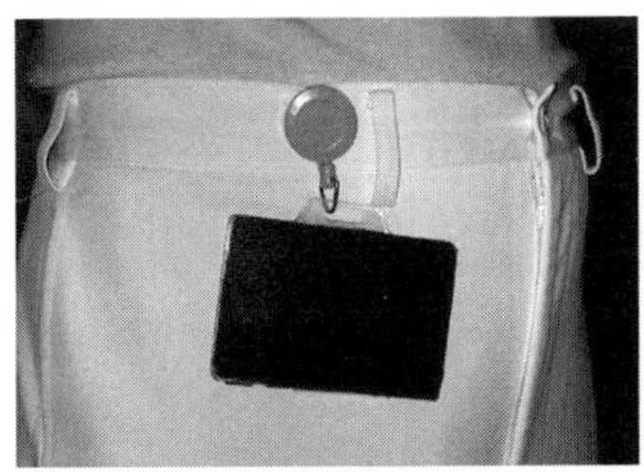

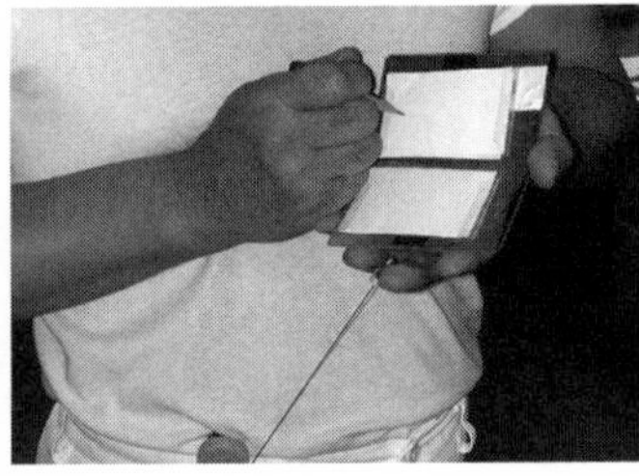

Figure 2-5 Waist-type memo-pad

2.5 Pin-type (Brooch-type)

This is a flower shaped leather pin with sticky-notes and a pen fixed to the back (Figure 2-6). You can simply see a reminder by turning it over after attaching it to the clothes with a clip. A nurse said that this memo-pad had reduced the number of times she scribbled notes on her hand. You can also use it by attaching it to your bag with a string (Figure 2-7). When you go shopping, you can easily look at the reminders without opening your bag.

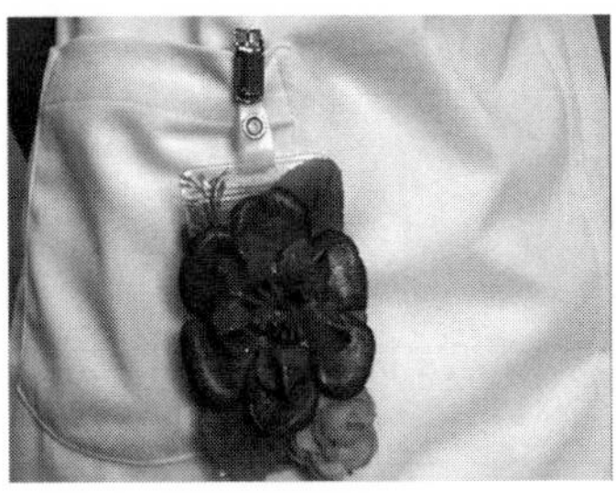

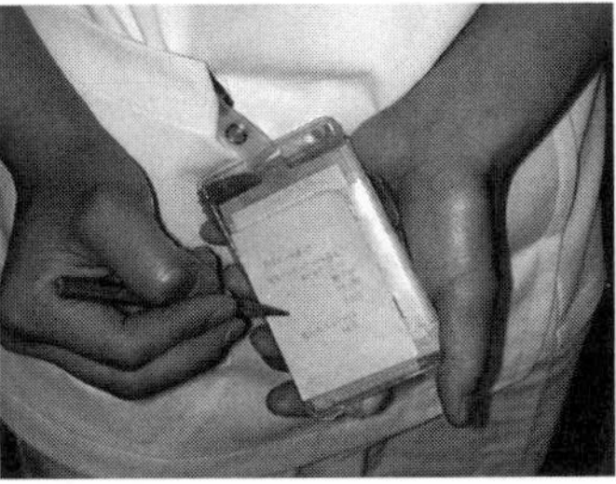

Figure 2-6 Pin-type (Brooch-type) memo-pad

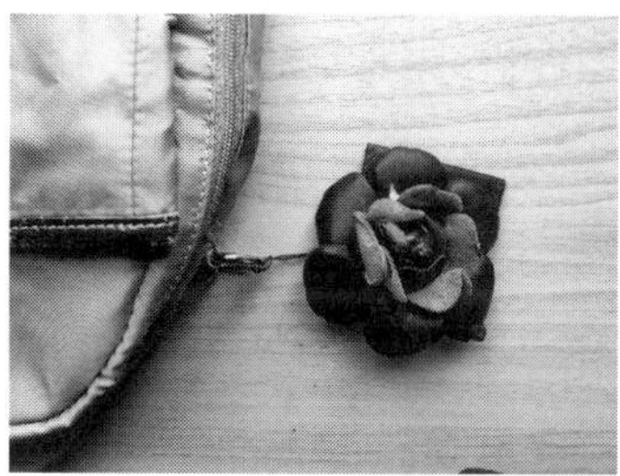

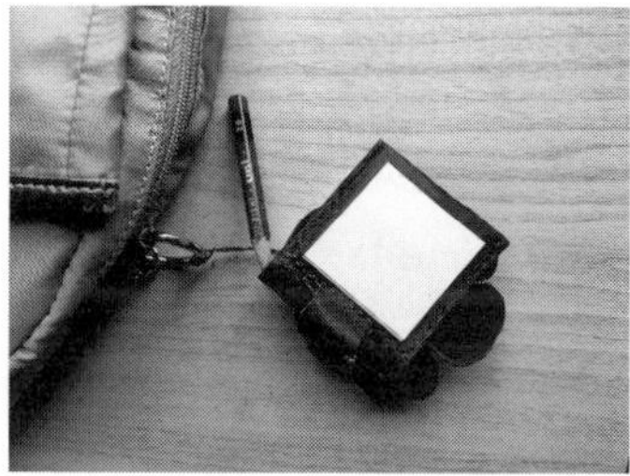

Figure 2-7 Pin-type memo-pad for attaching to bag

This prevents users from forgetting what they need to buy and what they already have at home.

2.6 Bolo-tie type

This is a leather bolo-tie (loop-tie) type memo-pad (Figure 2-8). A unique clasp for the bolo-tie is attached to the back to tighten or loosen the hanging cord. It contains sticky-notes and a pen which will appear by pulling down the front cover. More than 10 clients at the Memory Clinic have used it to write their shopping lists on many occasions. They could see their notes as soon as they needed to check them. If they do not like its swinging motion, they can attach it to the clothes with a clip. **The half-opening system** can also be applied to the bolo-tie memo-pad.

By the way, even if you write memos on sticky-notes, you often forget the memos. To prevent this, it is important to show a part of the sticky-note out of the memory pads. This allows you to notice the memos (see Figure

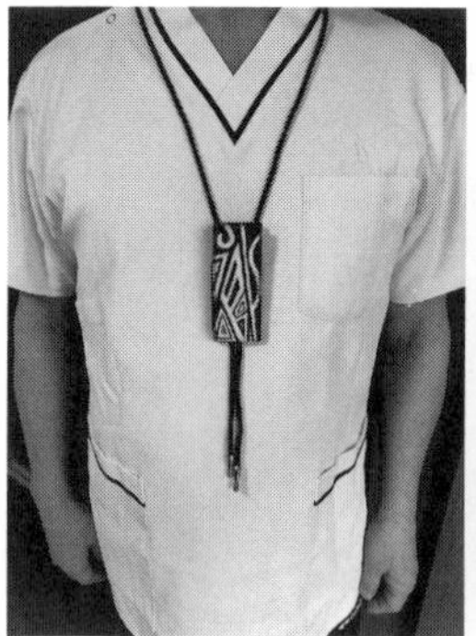

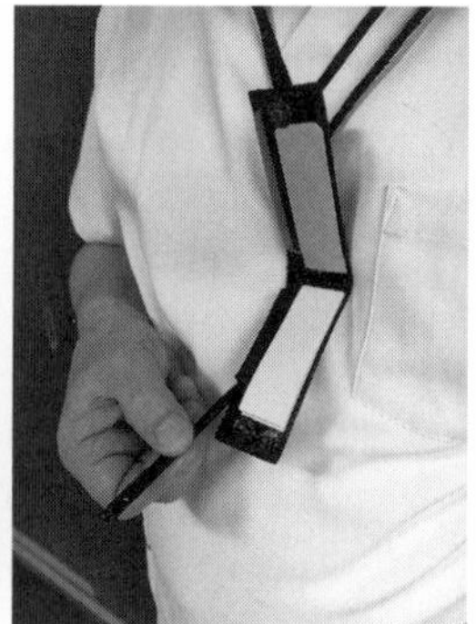

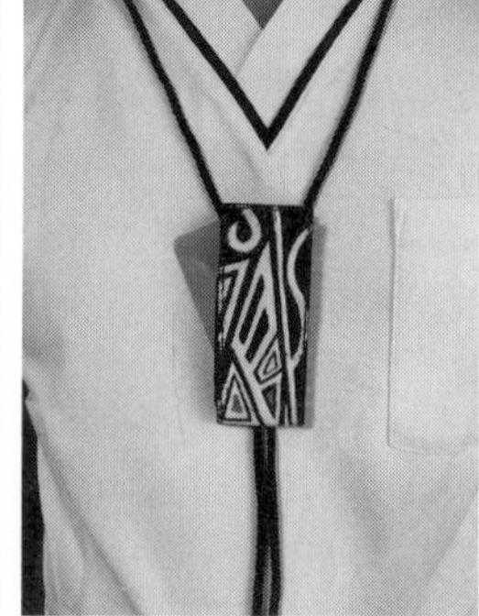

Figure 2-8 Bolo-tie type memo-pad

2-8 (right)).

2.7 Train pass-case type

It becomes difficult for persons with dementia to make payments with cash when their dementia becomes advanced. However, it has become possible to do shopping by using various cards. Thus, a unique commuter-pass case was created as a memo-pad, in which payment cards, business cards, sticky-notes, scratch memo papers, and a pen can be kept. Users also have a choice of placing it in their pocket or hanging it around their neck. Fortunately, it was commercialized by Kakura (http://www.kakura-shop.com/fs/netshop/ gr179/ls047abr) as Pass & Reminder-case (Figure 2-9). The user's name can be stitched on the leather case with an additional charge. You may give it as a gift, for example, to your parents when they retire or when you notice their minor memory problems. They may be happy to use the given pad and it will help them cope with their increasing memory problems. This is a train pass-case type of memo-pad that will be useful for any workers who commute by train.

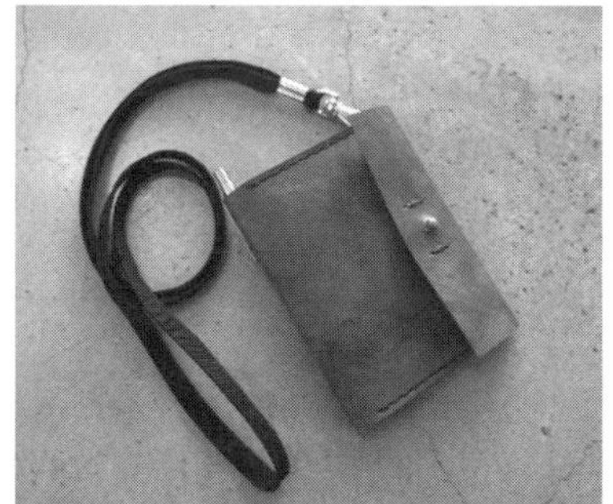

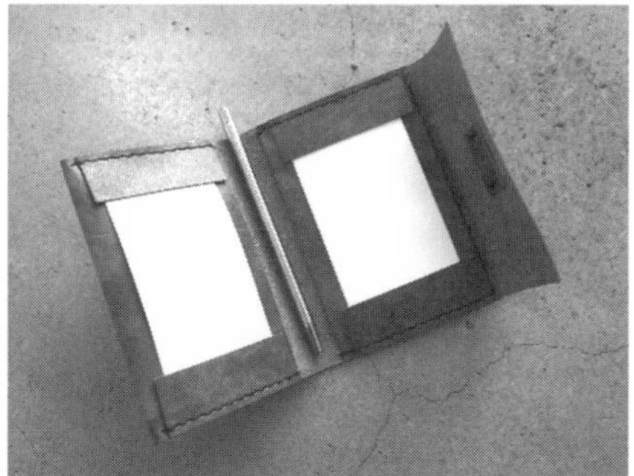

Figure 2-9 Train pass-case type: Pass & Reminder-case (Kakura)

2.8 Business-card type

This is a memo-pad which is made easily by modifying a business-card holder available at dollar stores (Figure 2-10). The manner of using it is the same as the above train pass-case type. It has a rubber string for hanging around the neck and a clip to prevent it from rolling laterally. By stretching the rubber string and touching the sensor of the cashier with the pad, users can make a payment if a credit card is included. A short string is also

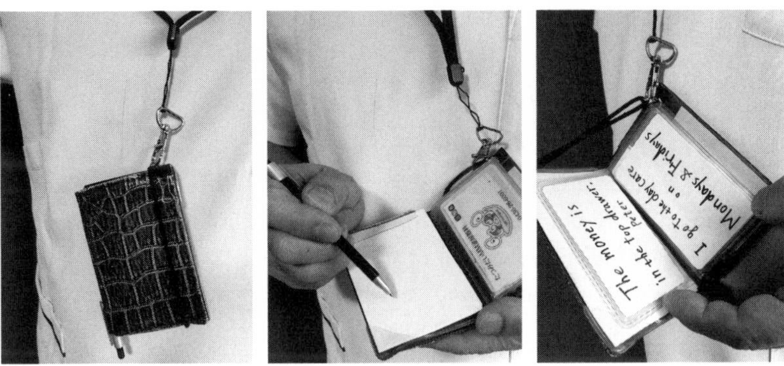

Figure 2-10 Business-card type memo-pad

attached for keeping the memo-pad half open. Family members can write down the answers to repetitive questions on sheets in the transparent holder of the inner side. I named this pad the "Smart memo-pad." This is easily handmade and inexpensive. Please check my website (search with "Kiyoshi Yasuda home page") to learn how to make these modifications. I hope that the business-card type memo-pads are also useful to normally aging elders who may be able to make these memo-pads themselves.

2.9 Hard-cover type

The memo-pads introduced so far require using both hands to utilize them, so they are not usable by persons with paralysis or who are already holding something with one hand. In order to make "**one-handed writing**" possible, a new style of memo-pad (Figure 2-11) was developed by replacing the mirror of a commercially-available compact with scratch memo paper and attaching a magnet to the upper edge of the compact. By opening the compact to the pre-fixed angle (approximately 135 degrees) and inserting the cover of the compact into the pocket of the user's clothes, users can write notes with one hand even while walking or holding luggage in one hand. Due to the hard cover, this pad is stable for writing, and opening the compact at 135 degrees is easier for writing than at 90 degrees. Persons with mild memory impairment can see, for example, a list of household tasks and check them off one by one if they leave the compact open all day long. Family members can also put sticky-notes on which the answers to repetitive questions are written.

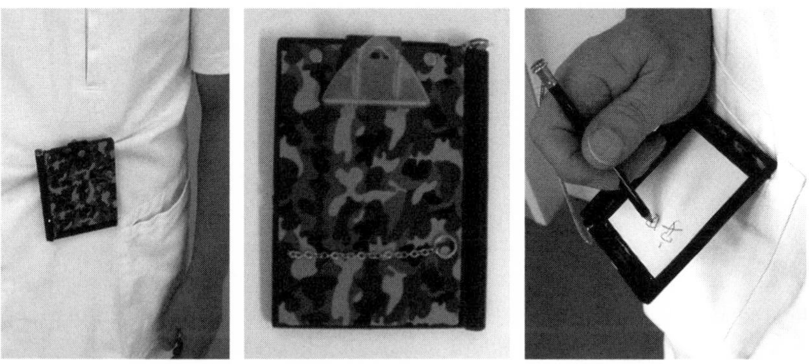

Figure 2-11 Hard-cover type memo-pad and one-handed writing

2.10 Summary of wearable memo-pads

In the coming years, the number of persons with memory impairments will steadily increase. It will be necessary for the elderly to change their old habits of "night writing" (waiting until the evening to update their diary) into "anytime writing" of diaries, in order to prevent them from forgetting what they wanted to write. They are also encouraged to use wearable memo-pads. The memo-pad shown in Figure 2-12 is made of high-quality leather made to motivate people to wear it as an ornament. I hope that many people will design such "fashionable" memo-pads and share their ideas on how to use them with others. Then, "literacy for dealing with forgetfulness" will grow among this group of aging citizens.

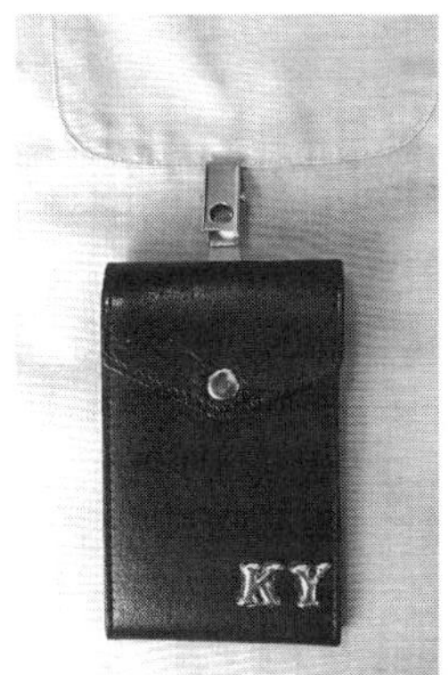

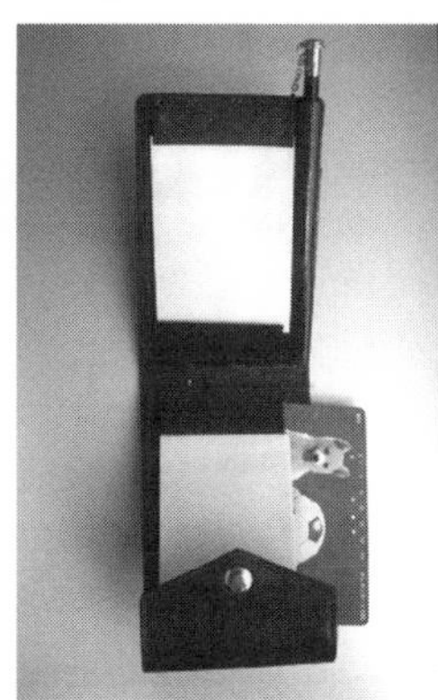

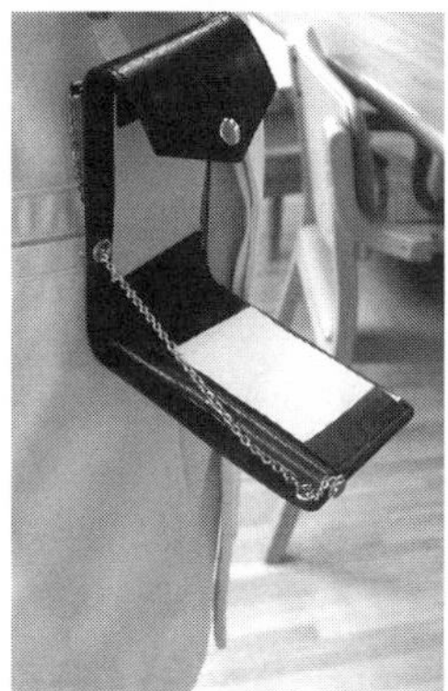

Figure 2-12 Ornament-like memo-pad

Most of the memo-pads introduced in this section were made and revised by Yoko Suzuki, Hitomi Miyawaki, Masayuki Ishi, and Furusawa Kawa Kobo. I sincerely appreciate their continuing cooperation.

3. Calendars and checking sheets

Persons with moderate dementia often find it difficult to write in diaries for several reasons such as "I am not good at writing," or "I cannot recall *kanji* characters." In order to deal with these problems, I recommended that they write down memos on calendars, as an alternative to the diary. Very few calendars suited for persons with memory impairment, however, have been available for purchase. Therefore, I have developed several unique calendars and check sheets. Copies of these are available from the section "Various calendars" on the English version of my website (https://gensoshi.jimdofree.com/home-pages-for-english/ or, search with "Kiyoshi Yasuda homepage").

3.1 Monthly memory-calendar

The most common excuse for being unable to continue keeping a diary is "because I keep a diary on a calendar, no need to write in the notebook diary." However, there is not enough space for the "diary" on the calendar since the space is for the purpose of noting appointments in a few words. To solve the problem, I created a "monthly memory-calendar" which has enough space for writing about daily events, in addition to appointments. In this calendar, space to write about daily events is hidden under the week

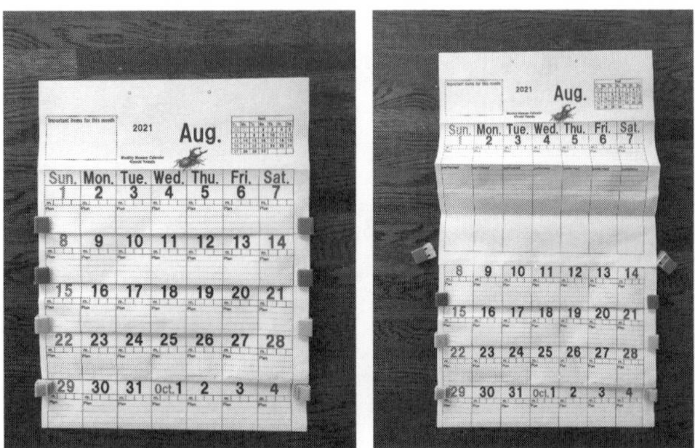

Figure 2-13 Monthly memory-calendar

row. At the beginning of a week, the user is to remove two clips on both the sides of the week to fold out the hidden space (Figure 2-13). The user is expected to repeat this process every week. OHOT's "*Slide Clipper Soft*" is recommended for the clip. You can find the original template for this calendar on my website. Making the monthly memory-calendar with the user's spouse or friends is recommended.

3.2 Half-monthly memory-calendar

The above "monthly memory-calendar is time-consuming to make. A half-month calendar can be made in a shorter amount of time. As the number of days to be presented has been halved, the space for writing has been doubled. It can be used with a normal calendar if a user wishes to see schedules beyond half-a-month (Figure 2-14). For elderly people who cannot remember the schedule for one month ahead, this calendar would be rather convenient.

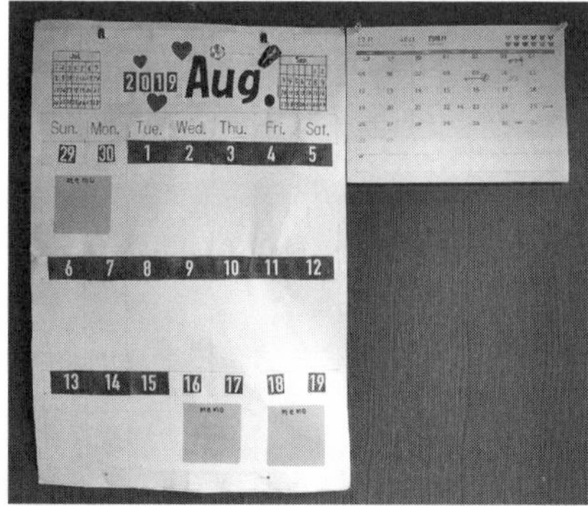

Figure 2-14 Half-monthly memory-calendar

3.3 Weekly memory-calendar

This is a weekly calendar with four to five sheets for each month (Figure 2-15). Each sheet has spaces for filling in appointments and schedules and writing about daily events. If the space is too narrow, users can write down on the back of the sheet. Punch holes on the upper-most side of the sheet so that you can file them together. Or you can hang it under a regular calendar available for purchase. You can print out the sheets from my website.

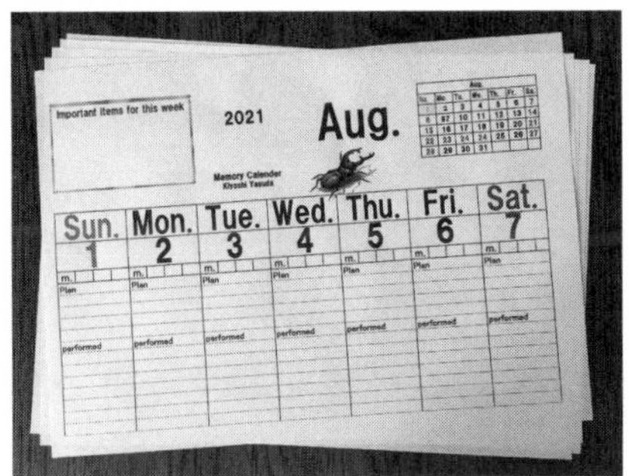

Figure 2-15 Weekly memory-calendar

3.4 Hourly memory-diary

As for daily events, persons with episodic memory impairment need to take notes immediately after an event they want to remember. To help with this, it is recommended that an alarm be set to ring every hour using digital devices such as a watch alarm, a timer, or a smartphone alarm (Sohlberg & Mateer, 1989). Then users can write down what happened in the last hour. A 75-year-old person with mild dementia succeeded to write an hourly memory-diary. The person was not in the habit of keeping a diary previously, but this system worked effectively for him. If a person does not remember why the alarm is sounding, use a recordable alarm clock or an IC recorder (see Chapter 3).

3.5 Schedule checking sheets

Persons with moderate-to-severe dementia tend to forget about the routine tasks they have to do, and the tasks they have already done that day. They may have things to do only on a certain day of the week such as putting out the garbage and going to the day-care center. For persons having these troubles, I created schedule checking sheets in which each day's schedule is written and the user is required to check the completed tasks one by one. As the example shows below, the user can also add his/her daily tasks into an empty space. There are various subtypes of the checking sheet such as the one-page-a-day and the half-page-a-day styles (Figure 2-16). Users can also modify it to a small-sized sheet and attach it to a wearable memo-pad. When attached to the pad, it will be possible for them to confirm the next tasks to be accomplished or the finished tasks even as they are walking to another location (Figure 2-17).

Date 20 Age Weather

To do in the morning		To do in the afternoon		To do in the evening	
Check the circle		Check the circle		Check the circle	
	O	Lunch	O	Dinner	O
Brush your teeth	O	Take medicine	O	Take medicine	O
	O	Wash the dishes	O	Wash the dishes	O
Take out the trash	O	Shopping	O		O
Get the newspaper	O		O		O
	O		O	Brush your teeth	O
Breakfirst	O	Afternoon tea	O	Bathing	O
Take medicine	O		O	Keep a diary	O
Wach the dishes	O	Bring in the Laundry	O		O
	O		O		O
	O		O	The fire is out	O
Hang the laundry	O		O	Door lock	O
	O		O		O

Day Day of the week 20 Age Weather

Free Memo

To do Task	
Check the circle	
	O
	O
	O
	O
	O
	O
	O
	O
	O
	O
	O
	O
	O
	O

Figure 2-16 Schedule checking sheets

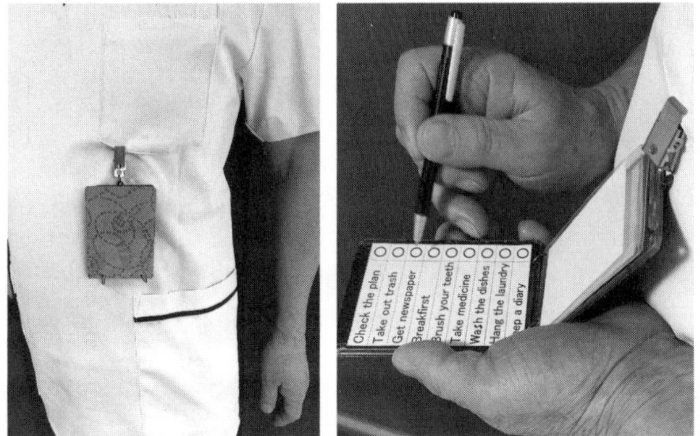

Figure 2-17 Portable checking sheet

4. Message cards and boards

Persons with dementia ask repetitive questions, such as, "Is it the day to go to the day-care center?", which annoys many family members. To address this problem, family members can write the answer to the question on a message card/board and direct them to read the answer. The effectiveness of "normal" message cards/boards, however, may often be ineffective for them. Therefore, I have developed the following special message cards/boards for those persons, for which you can find instructions on how to make them on my website.

4.1 MCI card

When a person with MCI is talking with someone for the first time, they do not notice that the person has MCI or memory impairment. Even if the

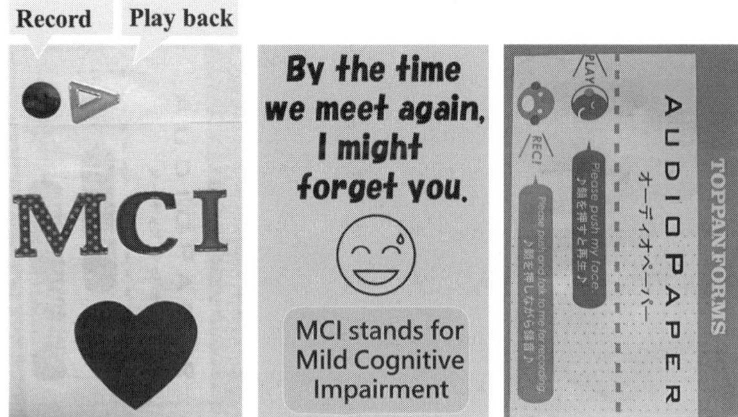

Figure 2-18 MCI card

person mentions it, they do not usually believe it. They will know, however, that the person forgot his/her face or the contents of conversation when they meet again. The person should show this card to them, for example, while passing a business card (Figure 2-18). The content to be written on the back side is freely decided by users. It can also be printed on the back side of a business card. The "*AUDIO Paper*" by Toppan Forms is inserted in the card. The 20 sec. message can be quickly recorded and played back (see Section 1.10 in Chapter 4).

4.2 Photo message card

Clinicians often provide written instructions to persons with moderate dementia for completing activities at home. However, they will often lose these documents when they go home. I created a photo message card on which clinicians attach a photo and an instruction; for example, the card could have a photo of the doctor with the message "Take a walk regularly." The card stands alone by folding its lower edge. Having the doctor's photo on the card seems to help them treat the card carefully and follow the instructions obediently. Family members can use a similar card to persuade them to go to the hospital or a day-care center (Figure 2-19). It may be more effective to place an IC recorder behind the message card with a recording of the doctor stating the message (see Chapter 3). The template of this card is on my website.

Bourgeois (2014) showed various kinds of memory wallet or reminder

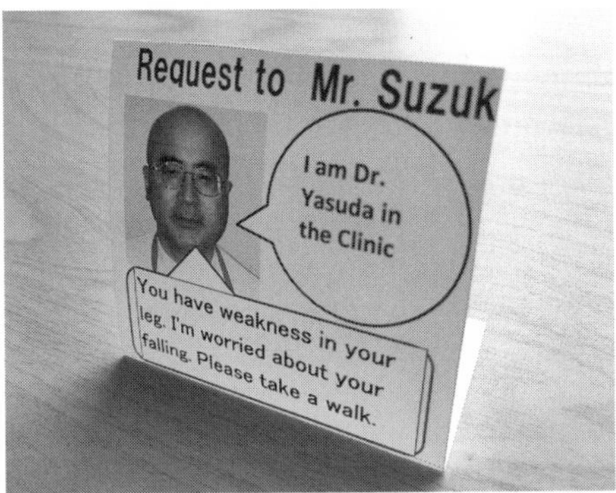

Figure 2-19 Photo message card

cards with a photo and a simple written message. Some cards can help prepare persons with dementia for their day at a day-care center e.g., "I am spending the day with friends," "I enjoy my time at Joe's Place," "The meals are delicious."

4.3 One-day message board

A whiteboard modified to stand on the table will be easily noticeable. Prepare small magnetic pieces to stick on the board for reuse (Figure 2-20). Write down the answers to repetitive questions on the pieces such as, "Today I go to the day-care center" (Bourgeois, 2014). They may erase messages on the board written with dry erase markers if the answers are different from their expectations. In this case family members could write messages with permanent markers on a sticky note. If they check off the items after the tasks are done, they can confirm them later. Putting favorite photographs

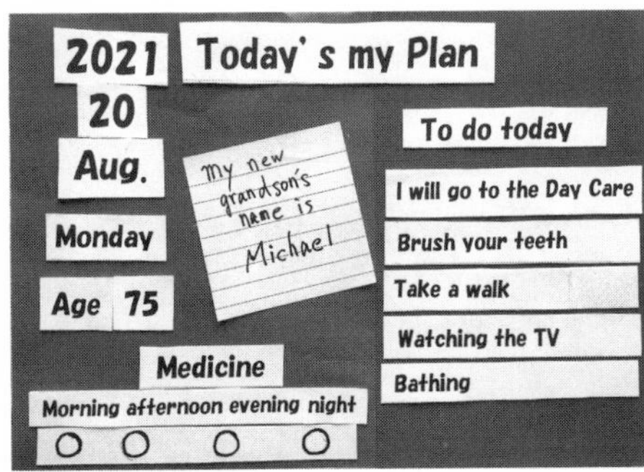

Figure 2-20 One-day message board

on the board may attract their attention to the board. If they still fail to notice the board, family members can put a device near the board such as a light that flashes when they approach or an IC recorder that emits favorite songs, or the voice of a grandchild, at specific times or regular intervals (as described in Chapter 3). It is recommended that family members direct them to the board to read the answer instead of giving answers verbally, with the expectation that they will learn to monitor the board voluntarily and find desired information before asking questions of others.

4.4 Cap-style message board

One of my clients with severe memory impairment was unable to retain memory for more than five seconds. For example, when she was informed "you are at ×× hospital now," and five seconds later when she was asked where she was, her response would be, "I am at the city hall." For such persons, we often put written messages on the wall or the door. Persons with visuospatial impairment, however, often fail to notice such messages. Therefore, I developed a cap-style message board. A written message card, "I am in ×× hospital due to a bone fracture." for example, is attached to the visor of the cap so that it dangles in front of her nose and she can read it whenever she looks up (Figure 2-21). To create this message board, attach thin tubes around the cap and under the visor, then insert a steel wire in the tubes. When you pull the wire out, a message card can be hung on the wire. The wire in the tube will not be visible, and the modified cap will look like a normal one. If you make this board by modifying your cap and try wear-

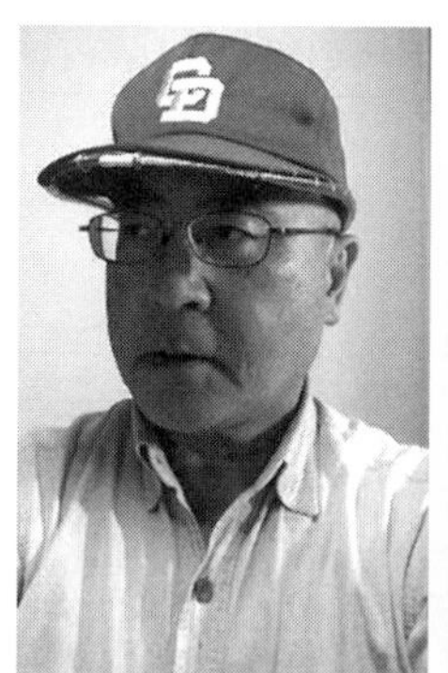

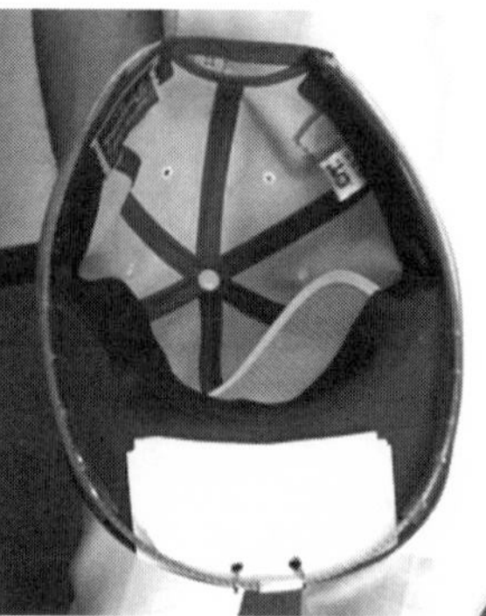

When the wire is stored

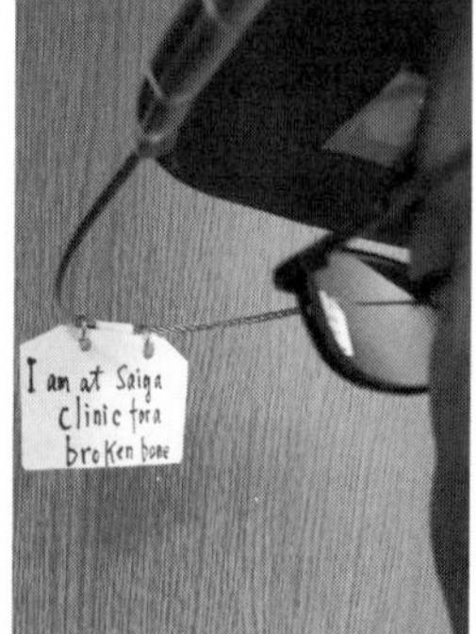

When the wire is pulled out

Figure 2-21 Cap-style message board

ing it, you will find it not so unpleasant to wear this cap because the message card is not as big as you would think, and the visual fields are not too restricted. Multiple cards can be hung from the wire at the same time. This cap may be helpful in managing repetitive questions on the same matter by hanging the answers on the wire. If you stack multiple cards, you can turn over cards to see other memos.

This cap was tested with the client above. While she was knitting, she seemed to think of something worrisome, and she raised her head. She noticed the message card, read it, nodded, and then went back to knitting. The message said, "I am in ×× hospital." This cap was also tested with a person with Alzheimer's disease who loved reading books. He noticed the message every time he looked up, and then he returned his eyes to the book and continued reading.

Sometimes both of them took off their caps, probably because they felt hot with the cap. Thus, a new and simple version of the cap was made with a sun-visor cap (Figure 2-22). With this version, a wire was attached directly to the peak of the visor. When users are eating, they can flip the message card (wire) up towards the top of their head.

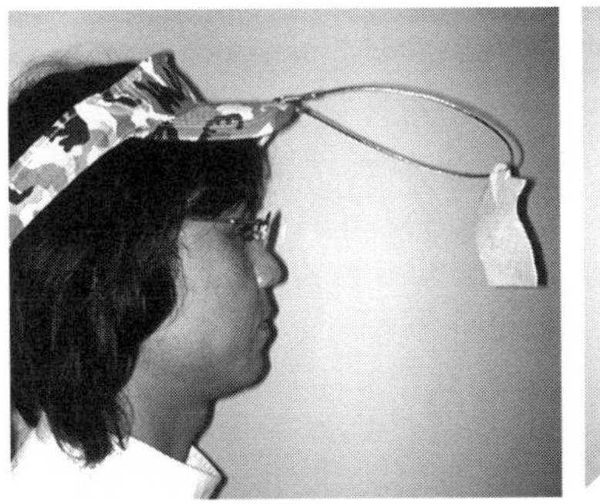

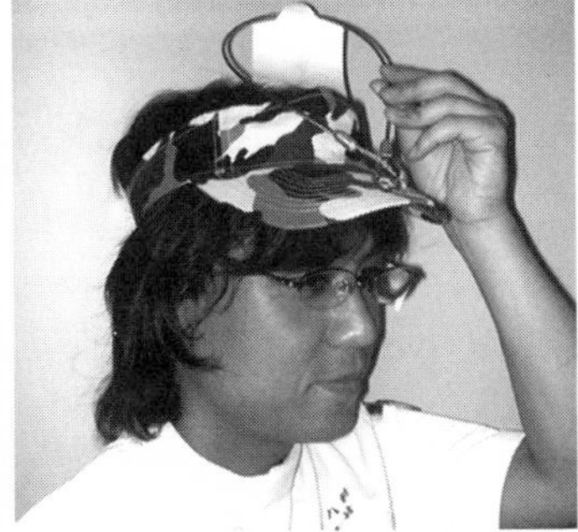

Figure 2-22 Sun-visor type message board

This cap-style message board at the person's nose can be applied to those people who have forgotten the faces of their family members. Persons with severe dementia sometimes ask their family members, "Who are you?" There is a case in which the husband of a person was locked out of his house when he went out to throw out the garbage. She had begun to forget the current face of her husband, although she still remembered his face from a younger age. In this case, the husband could hang the photo of his

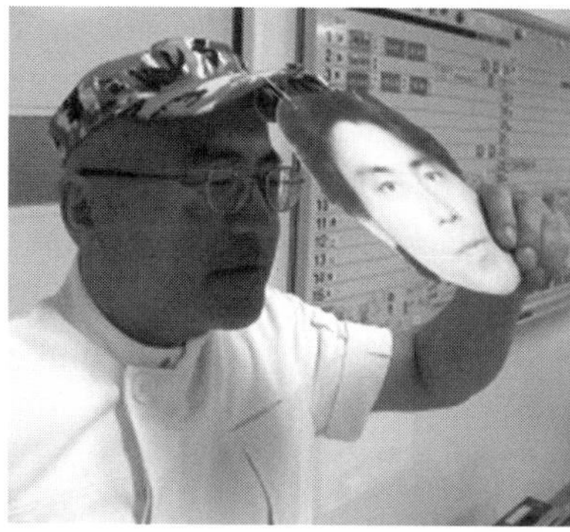

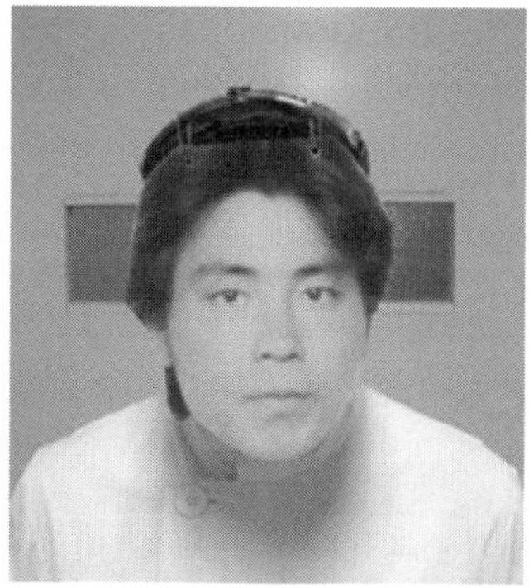

Figure 2-23 Hanging photo of younger age

younger self on the wire of his cap and show it to her every time when she approached him (Figure 2-23).

4.5 Chest message board

Another idea would be to have him hang the photo around his neck as a chest message board (Figure 2-24). It may be difficult for the husband to know which age of his face the wife recognizes, as her retroactive memory fluctuates. It may be his face in his 20's at one time or in his 40's at another time. One of the solutions is to collect his photos from the past to the present, sequence them chronologically on one sheet of paper and show it to her. It is recommended to have the wife select the photo of her husband from this array of pictures of him at various ages. She will most often select a picture from their younger years because of her preserved long-term memory.

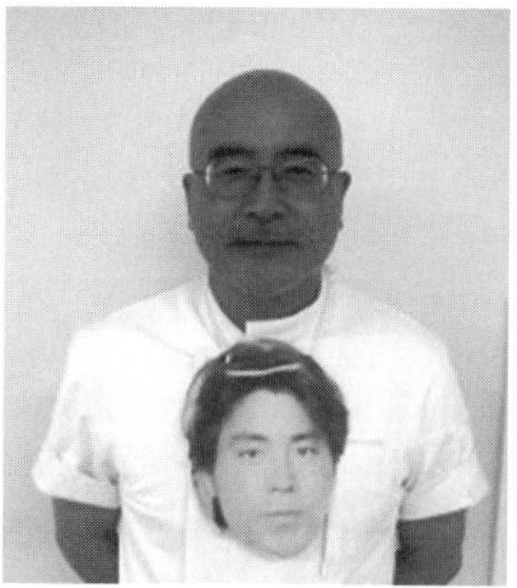

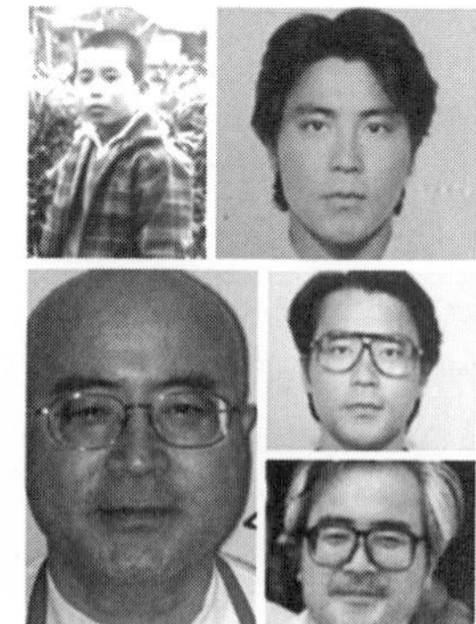

Figure 2-24 Chest message board

Bourgeois (2014) mentioned a chest message board putting 2 pictures side by side, labelled "My 25-year old husband," and "My husband now." This will show the wife that the two photos are of the same person. The chest message boards can also be used to manage repetitive questions. As dementia progresses, it may become difficult to compare the photos on the chest board and the actual face. In such a case, the cap-style message board may be recommended.

4.6 Neck and mouth message board

We usually speak to persons while looking at the face of the person. When dementia gets more severe, movement of the eyes becomes irregular and the visual field to which attention is paid becomes narrower. Even if the answers to the repetitive questions are written on the chest, it is possible that the persons will not notice it. Therefore, I made a face message board from two mouth shields on the market. The board can change its wearing position to neck, mouth, or forehead (Figure 2-25). Since this board will allow the answer to be displayed near the face, it may become one of the solutions to the above problems. In the future, electronic bendable displays will be able to show information. This digital message board will also be a beneficial tool for persons with hearing impairment because the speech of a wearer is shown as written text once it is recognized.

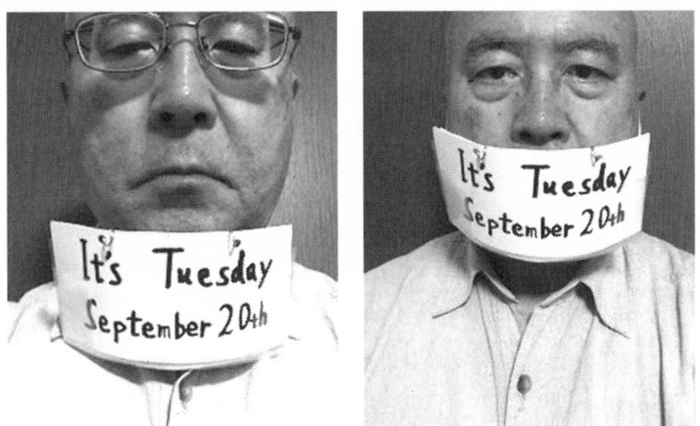

Figure 2-25 Neck and mouth message board

4.7 Compact message board

Section 2.9 in this chapter introduces a hard-cover type memo-pad (one-handed writing memo-pad) made of a cosmetic compact. In this message

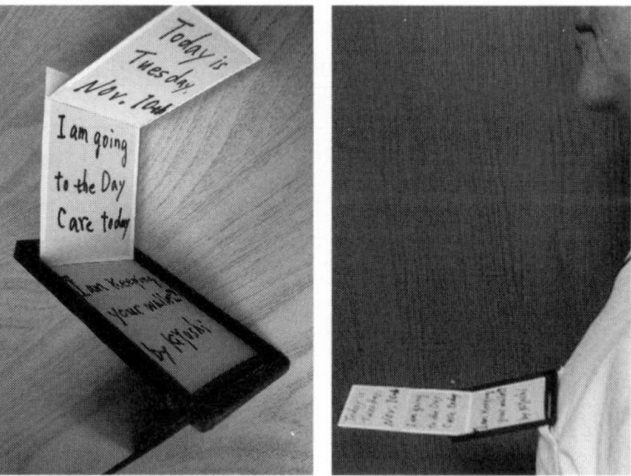

Figure 2-26 Compact message board: When sheets of paper are unfolded

board, the mirror was removed and a series of connected cards was put in the compact with one end glued to the compact itself. If you unfold the sheet, several messages will be visible in a row (Figure 2-26). This board can show several messages at a time. Some daily tasks such as shaving and cooking require multiple steps to be carried out. These steps are depicted on written reminder cards with or without illustrations (Bourgeois, 2014). These cards are shown to persons with dementia during the task within visual range for him/her to see while completing the task. However, when these steps are presented together at once, it is often difficult to remember for the persons. This compact message board can present all of the steps together or one step at a time in front of their nose as they engage in the task.

Related Topics —AT for children—

Some of the Low-Tech ATs sold for children can serve as a good reference for assisting the elderly. For example, a company called Addplus (https://www.addplus.jp/) sells products called a "Schedule Pocket" for hanging on the wall and "Let's go to toilet!" which shows the necessary steps of toileting performance through a series of picture cards. The company also sells a product called "Schedule folder to take with you." Bear in mind that the pictures used in these products are for children. You will need to modify them for use with adults in order not to insult them.

5. Supportive methods from other researchers

5.1 Supportive methods from a designer

A designer, Masato Yamazaki, cared for his mother who had dementia at home for seven years. He applied his knowledge of design to create "visual" Low-Tech ATs for her. For example, he designed and evaluated various message boards and posters appropriate for each stage in her development of dementia. He published a valuable case report that provided examples of long-term daily support by ATs for a person living at home with mild to severe dementia (Yamazaki, 2008–2009). Figure 2-27 shows a poster for identifying family members. Designers should be encouraged to create Low-Tech, Middle-Tech, and High-Tech AT.

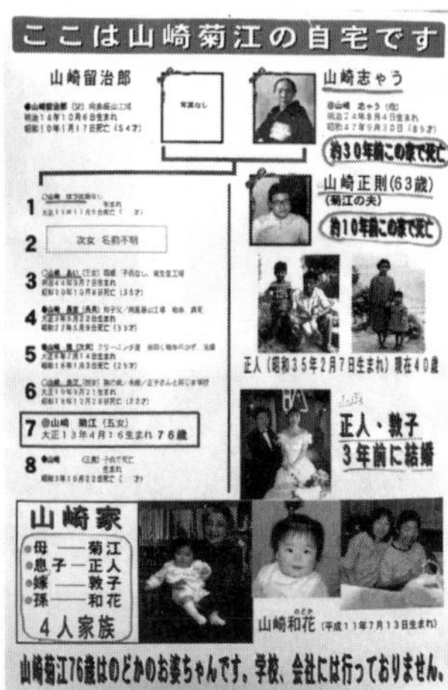

Figure 2-27 Instruction poster by Yamazaki

Related Topics —Creating environments suited for persons with dementia— Environmental modifications can be made to prevent persons, especially those with Lewy-body dementia, from having optical illusions. Some examples include changing fluorescent lamps, which emit flashing lights, to incandescent lamps, keeping the appropriate brightness in each room; eliminating shadows by removing hanging objects; removing stains from the walls; selecting curtains with no or simple patterns; and covering the LED lamps of electronic appliances with opaque tape (see Hickey, Bourgeois, & Brush, 2018 for more information).

5.2 Message boards and memory wallets/books

Bourgeois (2014) introduced memory wallets, memory books, and other Low-Tech ATs for residents with moderate dementia in care facilities. The memory wallets and books contain captioned pictures about familiar persons, places, and events that each user had difficulty remembering. Users improved the quality of their conversations by increasing factual statements and decreasing ambiguous, and perseverative utterances. Conversational partners decreased their use of questions and prompts during conversations. Figure 2-28 shows a magnet message board and a memory book used to facilitate communication. See Bourgeois (2014) for detailed descriptions. For reviews on other ATs, especially for residents in care facilities, see "Dementia and assistive technology (AT): Personal review" in the English version of my website (search with "Kiyoshi Yasuda homepage").

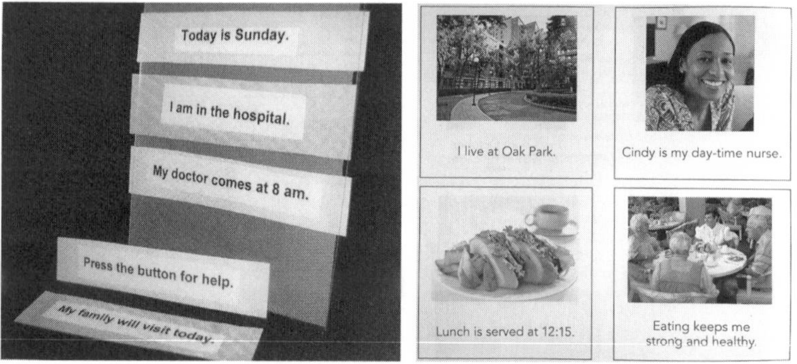

Figure 2-28 Message board and Memory book
Source: Bourgeois (2014).

5.3 Written cuing in response to repetitive questioning

In the study of Bourgeois et al. (1997), seven family members of home-dwelling spouses with Alzheimer's disease were trained to implement written cuing (index cards, memory book pages, or memo-boards) in response to repetitive questioning. Results revealed that trained family members were successful at decreasing repetitive questioning through written cues. In addition, intervention effects lasted for 16 weeks or longer and several family members reported successfully applying the cuing intervention to other nontargeted behaviors. Their efficacy in managing difficult behaviors of their spouses improved significantly at the 3-month follow-up assessment.

6. Diary *Tomorrow* for the healthy elderly

Although benefits of diary-keeping for persons with memory impairments have been well known, many of them find it difficult to do so. The New Memory Support Diary in Section 1.1 of this chapter proposed a format suitable for persons with memory impairments. It would be more beneficial to form the habit before the memory impairments develop because forgetfulness also occurs among the healthy elderly. Forming this habit, however, is not easy even for the healthy elderly. One of the reasons for this may be that the formats of many traditional diaries are inconvenient for them. Furthermore, factors such as how to handle or where to place a diary in order for them to easily fill it in and view it have rarely been addressed.

Recently, I have developed the Diary *Tomorrow*, which will be published by Escor (http://escor.co.jp) in Japan in 2022 (Figure 2-29). The diary has the following formats and systems which would facilitate diary entries by the healthy elderly.

- The double page spred of A4 size is set up for keeping a log for one day. Folding the diary into two, a user can carry a portion of the diary, a month worth or two, for example, at a time. In this way, the diary can be used as a memo-pad. At the end of a year, the user can bind them together.
- The right page is a wide blank space that can be used at the user's convenience. The left page is divided into many topics/items to fill in, which are important for maintaining the health of the elderly and for early detection of diseases (not necessarily needed to fill in all of them.) The topics/items to be checked include health conditions such as stress, physical pain/discomfort, forgetfulness, sleep, urination, bowel movements, and number of steps. Users can record meals, medicines and whereabouts of important documents and daily belongings.
- It is recommended that the diary is propped up against a copyholder at the corner of the table/desk. Transparent boxes containing stationery can be attached to the copyholder. A user may use furniture such as a chest of drawers for placing the copyholder if the table space is limited. In that case, the stationery may be kept in the drawers. The height of the

Date: Age: Weather:

Goal | Evaluation ○

Done	Time What to bring or event	Go out, domestic affairs, visitor, conversation, hobby, etc.
☐		
☐		
☐		
☐		
☐		

Meal content	Drinking water (coughing)	Done Medicine
Breakfast	mg	☐ Time
Lunch	mg	☐ Time
Dinner	mg	☐ Time
Snack or liquor, etc. ☐ appropriate ☐ many		☐

Health and information	
Condition ○ Appetite ☐ many ☐ appropriate ☐ few	Sleep (12, 3, 6, 9) Overall ○ Sleep onset ○ Total hour: Get up ○

Constipation times ☐ soft ☐ good ☐ hard Urine day times; night times

Body weight kg; Body temperature °C; Pulse white ( )

Walking steps; Gymnastics etc. time; Blood pressure (time)

Pain/stress	☐ no ☐ yes
Upset	☐ no ☐ yes
Forgetfulness	☐ no ☐ yes
Complimentary/reflection points	☐ no ☐ yes
Important things/text (electronic)	☐ no ☐ yes
Schedule, points to keep in mind	☐ no ☐ yes

Confirmation

☐ Key	☐ Pocket book	☐ Bag	☐ Locking	☐ Charging	☐
☐ Wallet	☐ Glasses	☐ Smartphone	☐ Discharge	☐	☐

Figure 2-29 Page of the Diary *Tomorrow*

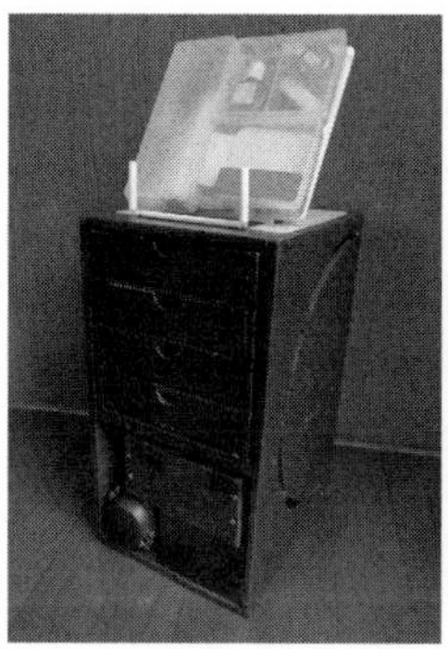
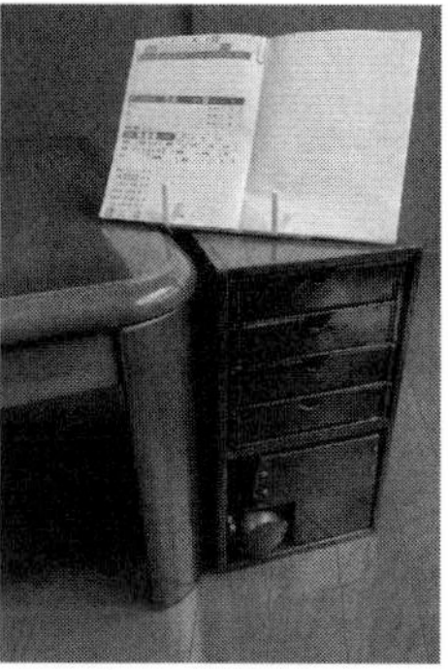

Figure 2-30 Copyholder with transparent boxes and a chest of drawers

chest and table had better be the same level. In this way, users can easily fill in the diary or view it (Figure 2-30).

- Some users may be interested in memory training while others may not notice themselves when a decline of their memory happens if not checked. This diary comes with a bookmark that can be used to hide parts of a page for memory training/check (e.g., hiding a section about past meals).

Electronic/digital diaries are already available on the market. However, paper diaries have advantages in ease of use and familiarity for the elderly. Furthermore, users can easily access information such as "to do list" while eating or watching TV. I hope the Diary *Tomorrow* will help the elderly keep a diary more easily. I also believe that it is beneficial for persons with MCI and younger people as well. If a user takes a photo of each page and uploads to the Cloud, it will be helpful for the users to search for a specific page later. Some users might want to put a PC or tablet on the chest for a digital diary.

6.1 Summary of Low-Tech AT

Clinicians often advise persons with memory impairment, MCI, and dementia to use memo-pads and diaries. These pieces of traditional stationery were, in fact, designed for healthy people. As a result, they find it difficult to make use of memo-pads and diaries. The fundamental problem is that only a few Low-Tech AT have been designed for them. In the current rapidly aging society, clinicians face increasing needs to develop Low-Tech AT which persons with memory impairment can use intuitively without much training. They, nonetheless, will forget how to use them and even the fact that they own them if they are not used regularly. They should, therefore, receive AT training. Users may need to be reminded to use AT through devices such as timers or smartphones throughout the day. It is also important for them to get accustomed to using the memory assisting ATs at an early stage of memory loss or at the healthy stage. In the last section, I proposed the new diary for healthy elderly and settings in which the diary can be used so that the elderly can easily refer to and fill in.

The Low-Tech ATs introduced in this book are easy to use, inexpensive, durable, and usable without electricity. Only 27 % of older adults with household incomes under $30,000 own smartphones in the U.S.A. (Dahlke & Ory, 2020). Recent estimates suggest that 58 % of persons with dementia live in low- or middle income countries (see Astell et al. (2019) for reference). Information on Low-Tech ATs would be useful for them.

Although instructions for making ATs are obtainable, developing them is not always easy. It took over 35 years for me to create the various Low-Tech ATs introduced in this book. Efficacy evaluations are not complete and will be continued. I hope that other professionals develop effective alternative memory and communication systems while evaluating the ATs shown here.

An engineer once said, “Low-tech products that work well will work even better if high technology is applied.” The bracelet-type memo-pad, for example, can be more useful if a smartwatch is attached on it. It becomes a hybrid AT that makes instantaneous recognition of memos possible along with other forms of digital information. The idea of cap-style message boards would suggest the usability and effectiveness of “smartglasses” which can show messages in the corner of the visual field. I am hopeful that the Low-Tech ATs in this chapter will open up possibilities for the development of new hybrid Middle/High-Tech ATs.

CHAPTER THREE

Supporting daily life with an IC Recorder

Prospective memory is used to remind yourself to do something in the future, for example to take medicines after meals, to call someone in two hours from now, or to do something specific at a certain time. The Low-Tech ATs introduced in Chapter 2, however, often fail to support these prospective memory tasks. This is because their main purpose is to log what the users have done, and not to remind the users of what they should do at a scheduled time. Although alarms that beep at specific times are efficient, persons with moderate/severe memory impairment may forget what they have to do when they hear the alarm. In Chapters 3–6, information and communication technology (ICT) devices available on the market will be introduced as assistive technology (AT), as well as examples of clinical applications. The AT devices that require electricity are called Middle-Tech AT (Drucker 2012). The first device I will introduce is an Integrated Circuit (IC) recorder. The IC recorder is the most effective device in assisting persons with prospective memory impairment and other challenging problems.

1. Experiments with the IC Recorder

1.1 Development of a voice-output memory-aid

Around 1990, I came up with the idea for a device that could record your message, such as "It is time to take your medicine," and automatically output it at the set times. Tadashi Misu of Chiba Institute of Technology and I spent seven years developing a Voice-Output Memory-Aid (VOMA) equipped with an IC chip. As far as we know, it was the first voice output

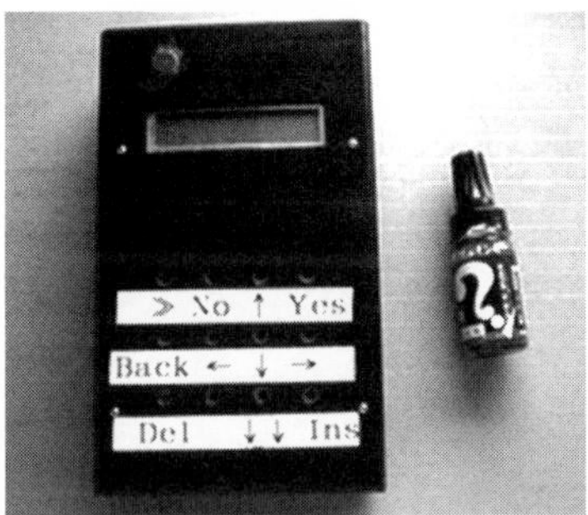

Figure 3-1 Voice-Output Memory-Aid

AT for memory impairment (Figure 3-1). With this device, you record various voice messages in advance, and then you input the times for outputting the messages. Persons with moderate/severe memory impairment might ask the same questions many times a day. To deal with this problem, the VOMA was developed to output eight different recorded messages up to 128 times a day, if necessary. Preliminary experiments were conducted on two participants with the VOMA using an A-B-A and A-B-B-A design to verify its efficacy.

During the first A phase (baseline), participants were instructed to do their daily tasks by their family members. Then, during the period B (the intervention phase) they were prompted by the VOMA to do the same daily tasks. Finally, during the second A phase (the VOMA was withdrawn) they were asked again to do the daily tasks by their family members. An examiner recorded the voice because their family members thought that their voice would not prompt the participants to follow the instructions.

Participant A was a 52-year-old man. He had language and memory impairments as well as hemiplegia resulting from brain infarction. When he was advised to do a walking exercise and a *kanji* letter writing drill by the examiner, he responded, "I will do so," but he did not perform them at all (A phase). However, when instructed by the VOMA (B phase), he exercised and recorded how many steps he walked and practiced writing *kanji* drills for 11 days in two weeks. During the second A phase, he began to forget to do the tasks, and after 24 days, he stopped doing the tasks completely.

Participant B was a 69-year-old man with Alzheimer's disease who expressed a desire to improve his memory. It was recommended that he do *kanji* writing drills. He did the task only for 6 days during the first 21-day period (A phase). However, he was able to do the task for 13 days during the next 21 days (first B phase) when prompted by the VOMA. During the next 21 days (second B phase) with the VOMA, he did the task only for 4 days. Therefore, the second B and A phase was canceled.

These results confirmed the positive effects of voice prompts from an ICT device for the first time (Yasuda et.al., 1999) although the experimental procedures were incomplete. According to the wife of participant B, he was surprised at the voice from the device and talked back to the device at the beginning. She said that as he got used to the voice he began to disregard the voice. This comment suggests the limitation of the "one-way" voice instructions and the need to develop a "two-way" interactive system in the future.

1.2 Utilization of an IC Recorder

Around 1999, Sony released an *IC Recorder* (IC Rec) with an "**alarm playback**" function. The function is almost the same as the VOMA mentioned above. Users can record voice messages, such as, "It is time to take your medicines," and set them to play automatically more than 100 times per day. It is also possible to set the messages to play by day of the week, such as "Today is the day to go to the day-care center" on Mondays and Fridays, and "Do not go to the day-care center today" or "stay home today" on Tuesdays and Saturdays. Additionally, messages for specific times and days can be set, for instance, "You will see your doctor at 10:30 on July the 7th." Family members are often worried that the other members with memory impairment will not be able to stop the messages or tamper with the device. The recorded messages, however, stop automatically. The function of holding is installed to prevent mishandling such as erasing records, changing the date, etc. The device works with triple-A batteries that last for several months.

I have used some versions of IC Rec by Sony (ICD-BX312, ICD-BX332, ICD-PX440) with more than 100 persons (Figure 3-2). Some of these devices are still sold on the Internet. The present version available on the market is ICD-PX240, which is 115 × 40 × 20 mm in size and about $50. In most cases, I recorded messages myself onto the IC Rec at the Memory Clinic, since many family members insisted that their voice would have no effect on the other members with memory impairment. After assessing what kind of messages each person and family member wanted to be output for supporting their daily life, the IC Rec with messages was lent to them. Approximately 20 years has passed since I started using this de-

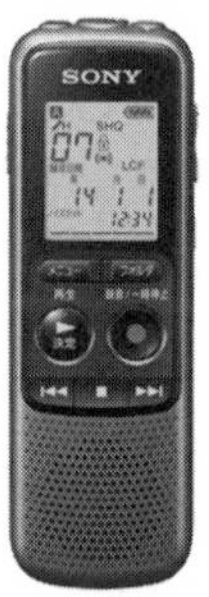

Figure 3-2 Sony IC Recorder ICD–PX240

Source: Sony Marketing, https://www.sony.jp/ic-recorder/products/ICD-PX240/.

vice. Almost none of the users lost the devices. This may be because they can locate the IC Rec device when they hear the spoken message. The users who were convinced that the IC Rec was useful in their daily lives returned the borrowed device and purchased a new one for themselves.

1.3 Experiments on the effects of the IC Recorder

The effects of the Sony IC Recorder were verified with eight participants (Yasuda et al., 2002a). These participants were persons who had developed moderate prospective memory impairments due to vascular diseases and brain injuries. When IC Recs were lent to the participants, they were wrapped with a piece of paper on which the following message was written: "Mr./Mrs. ××, please don't touch this device. From ×× of ×× Hospital" along with the examiner's personal seal. The message and seal were effective for all participants to remind them of why the device exists and to prevent them from moving it.

First, the examiner consulted with the participants and their family members to decide upon the messages to prompt tasks which each participant was expected to do and the time schedules of prompts. The examiner recorded a self-introduction and the messages with gentle tones and set the times of the messages to be output. Then, the recorders were passed to participants. The A-B-A single experimental design was applied to verify the intervention efficacy by the IC Rec (Figure 3-3).

The five participants (Par. 4–8) showed clear effects of the IC Rec. Each participant accomplished the tasks prompted by the recorded message, such as taking medicines, keeping a diary, doing vocal training, cleaning the house, taking a walk, reading notes to recall his/her own life history, and so

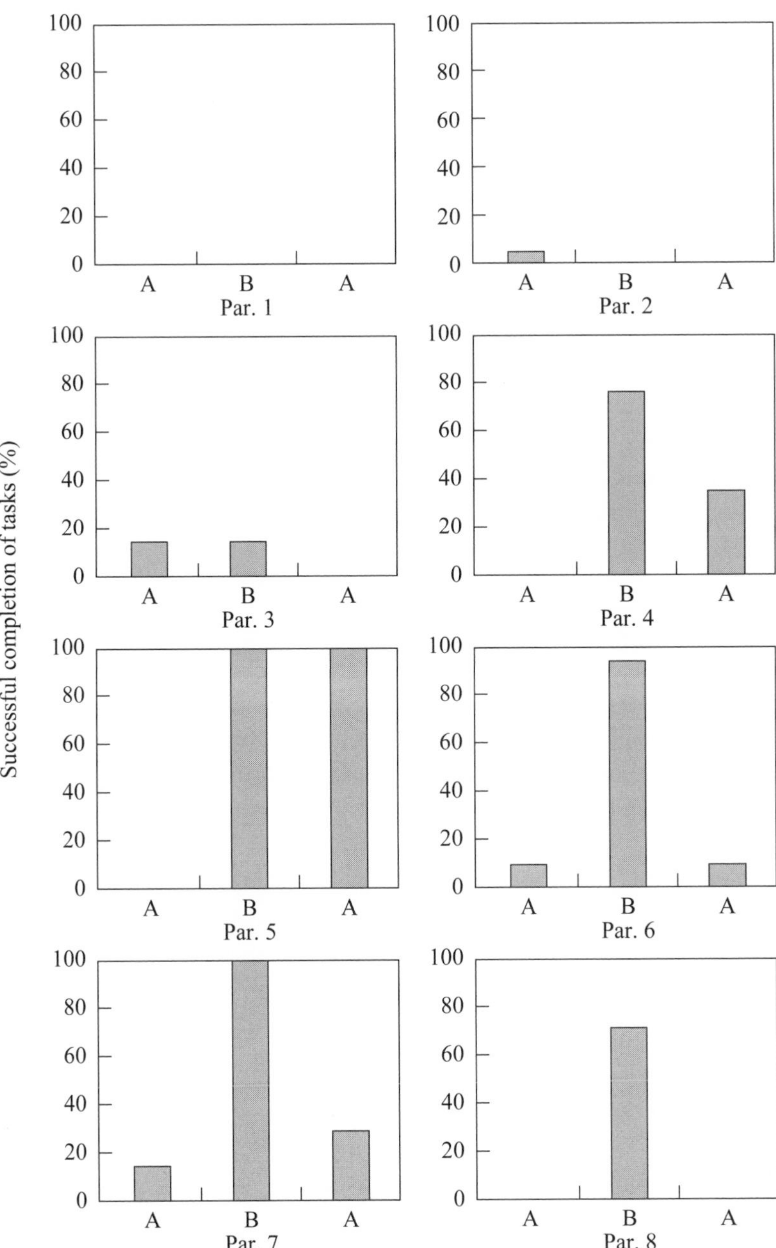

Figure 3-3 Results of experiments with Sony IC Recorder

Note: A = A phase (baseline), B = B phase (intervention phase: the IC Rec. was used), Par. = participant.

on. For a participant who liked to do gardening, the first instruction emitted from the IC Rec was, "Good morning. Please put this device in your pocket." By doing so, the participant could hear instructions while gardening. The percentage of task accomplishment for each participant ranged from 70–90 % (B phase in Figure 3-3).

After they returned the IC Rec (second A phase), the percentage of tasks accomplished daily decreased significantly for four out of the five participants (Yasuda et al., 2002a).

No intervention effect was found for the remaining three participants (Par. 1–3). Two of the three participants had subarachnoid hemorrhage, and the remaining one had a brain injury. All of the three had frontal lesions. During the study, those three participants were asked to do tasks such as, "Write in your diary" by the recorded message on the IC Rec. Instructions from the recorder, however, were almost ineffective. They took no actions saying, "I heard something coming from the device, but I was not motivated." Disfunctions in the frontal lobe often lower person's ability to initiate a task, which has challenged clinicians who work with these clients. Our attempts to facilitate initiation will be discussed in Chapter 6.

1.4 Feedback from family members

Family members can set their IC Recorders to have a beep sound before each recorded instruction. One of them said that the sound raised the person's attention level in advance before listening to the instructions. Some of them reported that hearing the third party's voice (the voice of "authority") through the IC Rec made the person more responsive and made him/her more punctual in doing these tasks. Many older adults often do not follow the instructions of their spouses, but they tend to accept advice given by their friends, grandchildren, and doctors. Family doctors would be happy to record their instructions. These experiments have suggested many promising uses of IC Recs as daily supports and these applications will be discussed in the next section.

2. Applications of the IC Recorder

2.1 Safety checks for gas, heaters, home appliances, etc.

There was a woman suspected of having mild dementia who lived alone. She was always worried about whether she had turned off the gas and heater after going out, or after going to bed. Then, the Sony IC Recorder (ICD-PX240; IC Rec) was set to automatically emit instructions to check them five or six times a day and the time just before going to bed. As a result, her anxiety about them almost disappeared. Today, there are smartphone applications or business services which can monitor the safety and environments of the home all day. Family members can also remotely operate gas, heaters, and air conditioners, etc. (as described in Chapter 4).

Another woman with dementia who also lived alone continued buying a lot of goods through TV commercials or catalogs, and consequently her living room was flooded with those goods. To solve this problem, she was given the following instructions from the IC Rec: "Your family members are going to buy the goods later. Please do not buy the goods now. They are also expensive." The message was given every evening when she usually had the urge to buy things. As a result, the number of goods purchased greatly decreased. Her family member asked the catalog companies to stop sending catalogs to her. It is also possible to block certain TV channels so as to prevent access to shopping channels. Family members can find instructions for how to do this by checking TV manuals, or searching websites. These cases illustrate that IC Recs can be quite effective for persons with dementia living alone once messages are recorded and timings of "**alarm play-back**" are set.

2.2 Supporting hobbies

The family doctor of a man with moderate dementia recommended that he continue his hobby of drawing. However, he drew only one or two pictures per month. As a way to remind him to draw more, the IC Rec prompted him "It is time to draw a picture. Let's begin drawing." Then, he came to draw over 10 pictures every month for about two years. (Figure 3-4). He forgot, however, what he was painting during the activity. For example, midway through drawing Mt. *Fuji* his drawing became very abstract. To maintain his focus on drawing Mt. *Fuji*, he could receive repetitive instructions such as "You are drawing Mt. *Fuji*" from the IC Rec every few minutes (as described later).

Calculation drills, *kanji* writing, and other kinds of drills are now popular as "brain-training" in Japan. It is more practical, however, to write your personal history, the names of friends and family members, and your age and address as well as the daily schedule every day. For example, a person with frontotemporal dementia, who had begun forgetting the names and

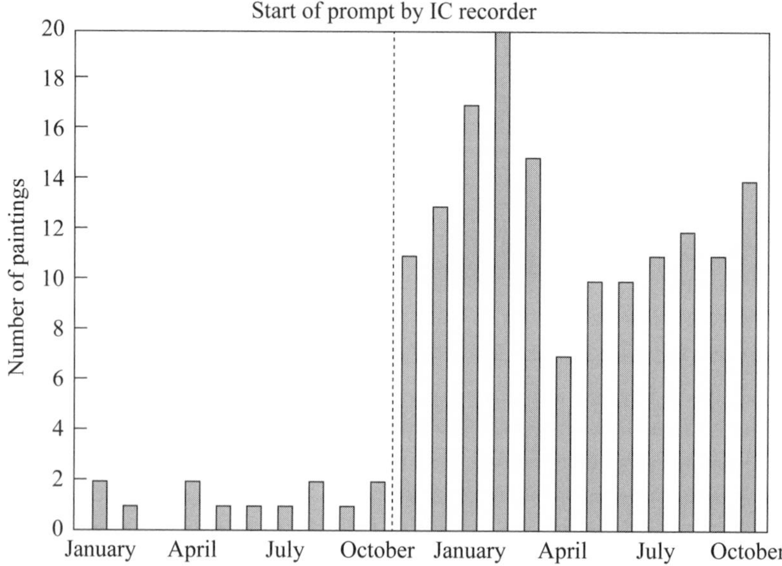

Figure 3-4 Number of paintings prompted by IC Recorder

faces of his friends, was prompted by the IC Rec to copy his friends' names written below each photo in an album. After this intervention, the person continued doing this exercise for a year. The IC Rec also prompted him to continue his hobbies such as an English conversation lesson, chorus lessons, and writing his personal history.

Related Topics —Clinical art therapy: Opening an art museum in the hospital—
Arts in Medicine programs is becoming popular today. In Chiba Rosai Hospital, the show space named "Rehabilitation art museum: *Asueno mado* [windows for tomorrow]" was opened in 1989 as the first hospital museum for clinical art therapy along the corridor walls in order to exhibit artwork by persons with physical and language impairments as well as dementia. A total of approximately 200 works had been always exhibited (Yasuda, Okada, Sadohara et al., 1993). Two persons, one with constructional apraxia and the other with arm ataxia, were unable to draw and write letters in proper form, respectively. They were advised to draw "abstract" paintings and write "avant-garde" calligraphy respectively. Persons with dementia were prompted to create art appropriate for their stage of dementia. For example, a woman wrote many letters as calligraphy on a wide sheet in the early stage of de-

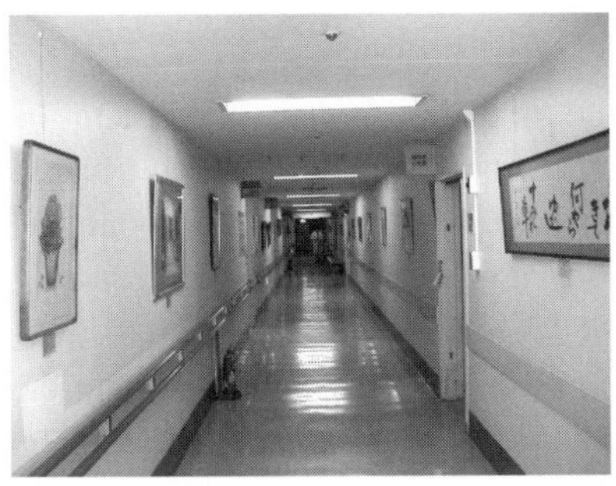
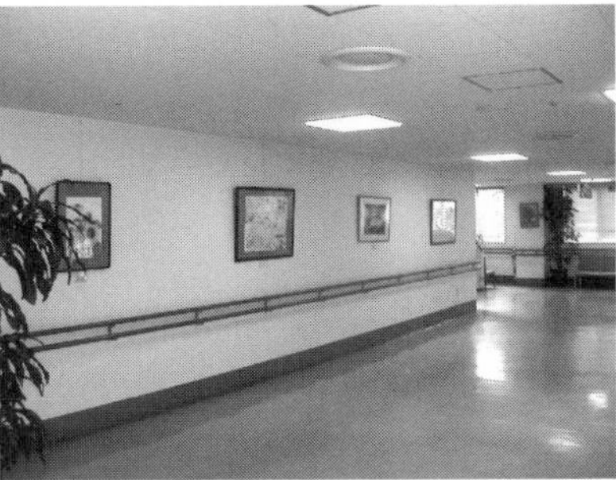

Figure 3-5 Rehabilitation art museum: *Asueno mado* [windows for tomorrow]

mentia. Then, she wrote a big letter on a small sheet in the advanced stage. Art-related activities, and exhibiting these works in public places, are thought to be effective for boosting the long-term self-esteem of persons (Figure 3-5). Regrettably, the hospital museum was closed in 2015, but a painting and calligraphy class for outpatients is still held outside the hospital (see Hickey & Bourgeois (2018) for arts interventions).

2.3 Prevention of getting lost

A person with moderate Alzheimer's disease tried to go out alone for a walk with his dog five or six times a day because he kept forgetting that he had already gone with his wife. There was also the possibility that he might get lost if he went out alone. To solve the problem, I recorded, "Mr. ××, you have already done your walk with the dog today. You don't need to go out anymore" on the IC Rec, and the recording was set to play automatically six times a day, the times when he tried to go out for a walk. This intervention completely succeeded in stopping him from going for a walk. It was effective for about one and a half years (Yasuda, 2002b). It was effective because every time when he began wondering whether he should go for a walk, the recording reminded him, "You don't need to go." This probably gave him some sort of relief. It can be stressful for family members to give and for persons to accept their instructions repeatedly. This is an example of **the strategy of providing information in advance**. Family members may ask someone for whom the persons have a feeling of respect to record instructions in a gentle tone. If this intervention works well, some of them may not need to lock the entrance door any longer.

2.4 Putting belongings in designated places

A family member of a person with mild Alzheimer's disease came to the Memory Clinic and said, "We can't find her bankbook and money because she changes the places where she puts them. We have asked the bank to make a new bankbook four or five times. Additionally, she began having the delusion that the bankbook and money may have been stolen by a thief." To deal with the problem, the following instruction was recorded onto the IC Rec: "Please put your coin purse in the top drawer. And please feel safe, because the door is locked to stop any thieves from coming in. Your bankbook is being kept by your son." This message was set to play several times a day. As a result, the person moved her coin purse less often than before, and she succeeded in remembering that her son was keeping her bankbook. This intervention prevented her from having further delusions of theft.

2.5 Prevention of incontinence

People are able to detect when their bladder is full and need to use the toilet. When this detection ability declines, toileting accidents happen, and with increasing frequency leads to incontinence. Several persons with this disability were prompted by the IC Rec every few hours to go to the toilet. As a result, the number of accidents decreased. Urine is pooled in the bladder at regular intervals, thus incontinence can be managed with this kind of intervention. To maintain the person's dignity, the IC Rec instruction to go to the toilet should be recorded by a third party.

There was a person with moderate dementia who forgot to position his body appropriately on the toilet bowl for defecating. He was invited to the toilet by the IC Rec message "Let's go to the toilet" at the usual morning toilet time. One minute later additional instructions, "Turn your body around," "Pull down your pants and sit down," were output. These successive instructions could guide him as expected, but unfortunately the defecation did not always occur since his bowel movement was irregular. This technology may be applied to prompt tasks with multiple and successive actions, such as getting dressed and preparing meals (as discussed in Chapter 7).

2.6 Returning the driver's license

Many elderly want to continue driving, even after they are diagnosed with dementia. Some persons with dementia get lost while driving. When they refuse the family member's advice to quit driving, this causes serious stress for their family members. Bourgeois (2014) showed an example of a written reminder card with photos of traffic accidents. A 70-year-old man with frontotemporal dementia drove his car at excessive speed and had an accident. Although his doctor convinced him to give up his driving license, his wife expressed her fear that, "He will forget that he was persuaded to stop driving by his doctor and will drive again." To deal with this case, I recorded a message of about 10-minutes onto the IC Recorder: "Driving a car is very dangerous for you now. If you have an accident, it may cause you or someone else to be injured or to die." The recorder was lent to his wife to have the person listen to it at home when he tried to go out and drive. This intervention succeeded in making him understand his situation. It is effective to ask someone whom the person trusts, such as his doctor, to record this type of message. In another case, I gave advice to the son of a man with dementia who did not give up driving. The advice was to tell his father that, "My car is broken, and I don't have enough money to buy a new car. May I borrow your car for a while?" Although the IC Rec was not used in this case, it could be a possible persuasive message to be recorded for someone else.

In Japan, the Road Traffic Law was amended in March 2017, and driving by persons with dementia became severely restricted. Early detection of abnormal driving by persons with cognitive disorders is done with a checklist to be completed by persons with possible dementia and their family members (*Anzen unten shien kyokai*, [Safe Driving Support Association] 2012). Any concerns revealed by this checklist should result in removing the driving license, and suggesting alternative modes of transportation. An electric bicycle, a three wheeled-scooter, or a senior car (a four-wheeled electric vehicle) are recommended. Except for the electric bicycle, they are covered by the Long-Term Care Insurance (see Sixsmith et al. (2020) for related information).

2.7 Prevention of repetitive questions

Many persons with dementia ask the same questions repeatedly because they forget that they have already asked them. Giving them a reminder note does not usually work because they forget the existence of the note itself. Family members sometimes suffer severe stress from their repetitive questions. Some persons have been known to use the phone to ask questions to others, and consequently the family members have to pay expensive telephone bills.

It took six years for me to come up with the following coping strategy using the IC Recorder (IC Rec) for the repetitive questions. We can use **the "repeat" function for the recorded messages** of the IC Rec. When persons begin to ask the same question repeatedly, his/her family members should roughly measure the time between the questions. If the interval is approximately 10 minutes, they should record the answer and have it played back every 9 minutes. This can be done through recording a message followed by 9 minutes of silence and press "repeat." For example, a family member might record "You don't go to the day-care center today"with 9 minutes of silence following the message, and press the "**repeat**" button. Then the IC Rec automatically plays the voice message every 9 minutes. They should stop playing the IC Rec when persons stop asking the same question. If persons tend to ask the same question all day, they can start this process at the beginning of the day. If the answer is provided every 9 minutes, persons may stop worrying about the topic and stop repeating the question. The point is to repeat the answer while persons still retain their memory. Family members could set the recorder to play at a longer interval if a person can retain the memory for a longer period of time. Use of rechargeable batteries is recommended because the IC Rec may have to be on for a long time.

If you want to repeat more than one answer at a regular interval, you can record several answers and silences as one set. For example, you can record "Today, you don't go to the day-care center," and record 10 minutes of silence, then record "Your son is keeping your bankbook for you,"and record 10 minutes of silence. In this example, you can make a 20-minute set with two messages and repeat it. The next day, the family member just has to press the repeat button since the above recordings are left on the IC Rec. Practical examples will be introduced later in this section.

In many cases repetitive questions tend to occur at specific times of a day; for example, a person may say "Is today the day to take out garbage?" every morning, or "I would like to go home" every evening. In such cases, a family member should prepare several sets of recorded messages and play each of them at a specific time. Since this method requires him/her to press the "repeat" button, it cannot be applied to persons living alone. Instead, a family member living away can record all the messages and set the time for automated "**alarm play-back**" for each message. This may sound time-consuming but once this is done, these messages will be automatically played and the family member just has to come and change the battery every now and then. Recently, a method for managing repetitive questions using a smart speaker through remote control became available as described in Chapter 4.

Family members are sometimes worried that persons may find the repeated messages annoying. There is usually no need to worry about this. Many persons who adopted this intervention did not remember, for example, what they had heard 10 minutes ago, and thus every time they hear the message they appeared to feel as if it was the first time. Family members have been also concerned that the recorded messages will be annoying, but it did not take long for them to get used to the recordings and to start ignoring them.

There was a person with dementia who was released from the hospital with a urinary catheter. Because he forgot the reason for the catheter, he attempted to pull it out almost every 10 minutes, and his family members had to take turns watching him 24 hours per day. For this person, the message "Please don't pull out the tube for your urinary problem" was recorded and played every 10 minutes by the method mentioned above. One of them reported that "the number of attempts to pull out the catheter noticeably decreased."

A person with a gastrostomy tube protested to his wife every day asking, "What is this? Why can't I eat food?" The detailed answers were recorded and repeatedly output for him from the IC Rec. As a result, he stopped pulling out the tube. The repetitive questions may be resolved by **the strategy of providing information in advance**, recording the message and using the repeat function of the IC Rec.

2.8 Recording long explanations

Persons with MCI or mild memory impairment cannot memorize long explanations. For example, they cannot retain an explanation given by their doctor about diagnoses, or by agents of insurance companies about their pension system. The IC Rec's recorded message strategy may be useful for them. Recorded explanations can be listened to repeatedly at home. A clerk in her 30's at a hospital had developed memory impairments after a car accident and had to resign her job because she was unable to remember the updated procedures for medical insurance. Memory tests showed that she had difficulty in retaining the contents of stories over three minutes. As a therapeutic training strategy, I recommended that she record several news stories from the TV every morning, listen to them, and write them down repeatedly. One purpose of this training was to help her recognize her deficit in memorizing stories and form the habit of recording information onto an IC Rec. If such persons recorded new information at work, listened to it, summarized it in a notebook at home, and looked at the notebook when they were trying to remember the information, they might ask his/her co-workers fewer questions. If this is a successful strategy for them, they might be able to return to their previous job.

An officer in his 40's had a car accident and sustained multiple injuries including memory impairments. He returned to his old job, but was transferred to a new department. He could not remember the new job procedures or daily instructions. I recommended that he hang the IC Rec around his neck, take notes about the instructions given every morning and then record messages about the instructions. This allowed him to listen to the information that he could not remember even by looking at the notes. Meanwhile, he input the schedule for the following day into a small personal computer (PC). He started up the PC every morning, erased each task in the schedule once it was completed, and then moved on to the next task. After coming home, he transferred the recorded information on his IC Recorder to the PC. He said that the voice recording was helpful because he could hear the emotions of the speaker on the recording. He listened to the recording by using the repeat button.

A pen-type voice recorder "Penvoice S" by GLORDGE can record voices simultaneously while taking notes with a pen. Recent smartphones can transcribe spoken messages into text messages but their accuracy is often imperfect.

2.9 Failures with IC Recorders

A person with mild dementia visited a barber at the end of the year, and was asked to come back in the new year because the barber was fully booked. He was not able to retain this information so he kept returning to the barber before the new year. As a solution, the information "Let's go to the barber the next month in January" was recorded onto the IC Recorder and played for him. However, he got angry, saying "I don't want to be controlled by this device" (Yasuda, 2002b). This could easily happen when someone is already convinced of an idea. For them, the IC Rec may not be the best way to convey this information. I should have asked the barber to give him a reservation card for a specific day in the new year. This episode suggests that **the strategy of providing information in advance** using recorded messages may not be effective for all persons. We always need to provide the strategy that the person will accept. Another idea is to record instructions on the IC Rec accompanied by the individual's favorite music (see Chapter 6).

2.10 Summary of IC Recorders

Yasuda et al. (2002b) reported that when a man with Alzheimer's disease listened to the instructions by the IC Rec, he sat up straight and fell to his knees before the IC Rec. After listening, he courteously bowed to the IC Rec, saying "Thank you very much for your kindness" and asked his wife "Is the person inside of this device?" Although his response may seem strange, it gives us valuable insights. When voices come out of the device, he did not regard the IC Rec just as a recording device, but rather as a box in which a small person exists.

In the old days when electric cables appeared in the Japan for the first time, some people thought an extremely small person was running inside the cables. More recently, persons with dementia have been observed talking to the photograph of an actor/actress printed on a poster, or newscasters on the TV monitor. It is, therefore, understandable that the person bowed to the IC Rec that spoke. When I heard of the above episode in 2000, I realized the profound implications of the efficacy of using ICT devices with persons with dementia (Yasuda et al., 2002b).

In many cases, when family members are first advised to use the IC Rec, they were skeptical and said, "he/she cannot control the device by himself/herself." This turned out not to be an issue once the IC Rec was set up and messages were recorded, since the messages were played automatically. There have been some examples of failure, but it was successful in 60–70 % of the persons with mild and moderate dementia. If written instructions are not adequate for a person, voice instruction should be tried. The effects of this method or any methods to manage dementia will need to be continuously monitored and modified if necessary, as the disease develops over time.

The efficacy of using the IC Rec was documented in Yasuda et al. (2002a; 2002b) but replicated only by Fujita et al. (2009). More professionals need to have the knowledge of such a useful device. They should learn how to operate the device, design an evaluation procedure, and explain it to their clients and the family members. Even young family members could easily learn to operate and set up the IC Rec in order for the persons to utilize it.

As of March 2021, there is another version of the IC Recorder, ICD-TX650 by Sony. This slim pen-type recorder also has the "**repeat**" and "**alarm play-back**" functions. Elderly people, however, may find it too small to handle, and the volume of the voice output seems to be too low for them. For the older users the ICD-PX240 by Sony was recommended. When the sound of the IC Rec is too low, a small speaker can be used to increase the volume. There are many other IC recorders produced by other companies. **However, most of them do not have the "alarm play-back" function**.

A product called "*Seikatsu* [life] call" by Technos can output a recorded voice at a pre-set time. A unique function of this device is that it will link to the remote family member if the user yells out loudly. Recently, several IC voice recorders that can continue recording up to one month became available. In addition, most of them will detect a voice and start recording automatically even if a user forgets to press the record button. A user can bring it to places where he/she is likely to receive a long explanation or instruction. "*AutoMemo*" by SOURCENEXT is a voice recorder that automatically converts recorded audio files into written texts, and transfers the texts to smartphones or PCs.

Some application programs on smartphones can also be equipped with an "**alarm play-back**" function. Compared with these devices and programs, the Sony IC Recorders are small, handy, and inexpensive. The battery lasts for a long time; the quality of the sound is good; and the output stops automatically, all of which are helpful and usable for the elderly. Therefore, the IC Rec is the most useful Middle-Tech AT currently available. The IC Rec, however, was not designed for persons with memory impairments. Several functions need to be drastically revised for maximum useability. Engineers and programmers will utilize our experiences introduced in this chapter before developing new and more effective Middle-Tech ATs for persons with dementia.

CHAPTER FOUR

Commercially-available communication and information devices

Commercially-available communication and information devices that require electricity are defined as Middle-Tech AT in this book. The Sony IC Recorder (ICD-PX240; IC Rec) was described in Chapter 3. In Chapter 4, various Middle-Tech ATs are introduced. Some Low-Tech ATs such as stationery, toys, games, and stuffed animals are also described in this chapter. Japan has the most aged population so that many products for the elderly are on the market. Some of those are likely to be unknown in other countries. Please look for similar products in your country.

Persons with MCI or dementia and family members may find it difficult to set up Middle-Tech ATs due to difficulties in understanding the manuals. Recently, shops that sell these products are offering in-home services. Alternatively, users can get advice remotely over the Internet or telephone. These services are important to get them started and continue using Middle-Tech AT. Some products or functions can be replaced with smartphone application programs (apps) which will be described in Chapter 5.

1. Devices for information management

1.1 Notice sticky-note, posters, and wrist-bands

Recently, several "stand-alone" sticky-notes have become available for sale. Messages are easier to see when the note is standing on the desk than when it is lying on the desk. If a "To Do" list is on the stand-alone sticky-note on the desk, it is likely to be helpful in reducing the number of forgotten tasks. I found one of these stand-alone "To Do" sticky-notes called "*Lightia*" by

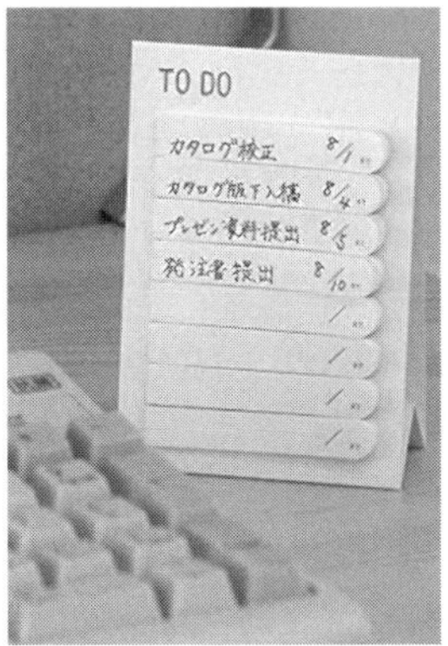

Figure 4-1 Sticky-note "Lightia"

Note: Each line can be peeled off separately.

Source: Sun-Star Stationery, https://www.sun-star-st.jp/campaign/standard_stationery/lightia/index.html.

Sunstar Bungu very convenient: there are eight lines on each sheet and each line can be peeled off separately. A user can peel a line off after the task on the line is completed.

Family members often use a notice poster on the wall to organize information. As persons with dementia often have impaired visuospatial attention, they may fail to notice the posters. One solution for this problem is to decorate the perimeter of the poster or memo-board with electric lights. A neon string called "*neon fiber*" is sold by several companies. A neon wrist-band called "*Clip-on marker*" by Niteize has blinking LED lights powered by button batteries. Messages can also be written on the surface of the wrist-band.

1.2 Memo-stand for medications and medication dispensers

Persons with dementia forget to take their medicines more often than they think they do and some forget the reasons why they take the medicines prescribed by their doctors. Figure 4-2 is a desk-top memo-stand designed to attract persons' attention and to remind them of the reasons for medications. This stand is made from a milk carton. Two sides of the stand can list messages from their "doctors" and "grandchild." The other two sides may list information about prescribed medicines and the schedule for taking medicines. The original template of the stand can be printed from my website (search with "Kiyoshi Yasuda homepage"). The medicine envelopes

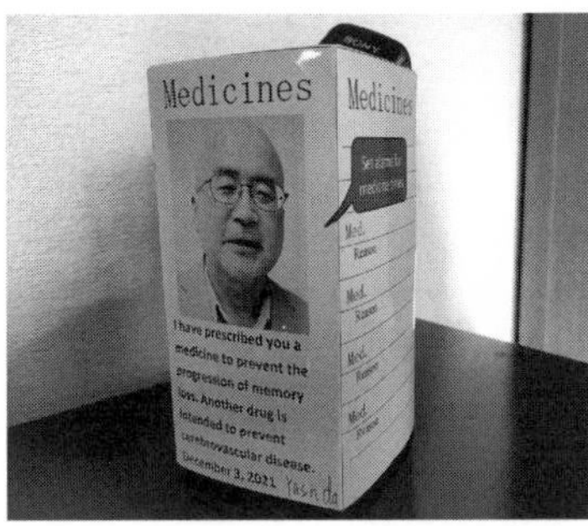

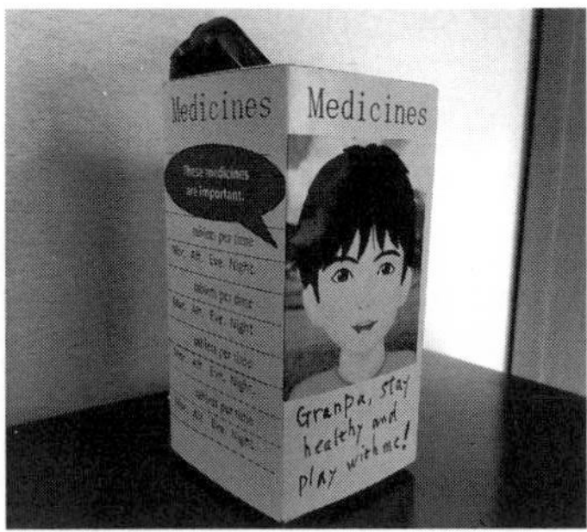

Figure 4-2 Desk-top memo-stand for medications

could be placed inside of the stand as well as the Sony IC Rec. If the alarms or voices by the IC Rec are set for automatic output, it will be more effective to prevent the persons from forgetting (see Chapter 3).

Pill cases, pill calendars, and medicine dispensers are available on the market. For example, "*Okusuri Hausu* [medicine-house] *series*" by Warm Heart is a calendar which has many small pockets for medicines, for one day, one week, or one month. The IC Rec can be hung on the calendar to remind users when to take their medicines.

Electric medicine dispensers are a type of pill case that sounds an alarm when it is time to take medicines. These are readily available on the market and are reasonably priced. Search for them on the Internet with following keywords of "pill box with alarm" and "pill dispenser." There are single day pill cases to use when out of the house. There are different sizes of each pocket of the pill case to accommodate few or many pills. Nevertheless, if you cannot put all of the medicines into the pockets, detach the alarm device from the pill case if possible and put it beside the pill box with big pockets.

A one-week pill box called "*Kusuri* [medicine] *Call*" by Technos will signal users to take a medicine with sounds and lights (4 times a day). This device can also output recorded voice messages, such as "Have you had a meal?" Another product, "*Okusuri Nondene* [take your medicines]" by Ueshima Denkosha, is a device that pops out a medicine case at set times. A device called "*Fukkun*" by Ishigami Seisakusho is designed specifically for users at care-facilities, and a medicine package for each user pops out at set times. If users forget to take the medicine, the incident will be reported automatically to their family members by mobile phone. In other cases, you could also ask visiting pharmacists to keep an eye on whether users are taking their medicines properly.

1.3 Location of personal belongings

Wireless tracking tags can be attached to belongings that are often lost; pushing a button on the main unit causes a sound to be emitted from the tag attached to the belonging. For example, you attach a tag to your wallet, and if you press the button for the wallet, the tag emits a sound. An example of this device is the "*Key Finder*" by Foxnovo that comes with a set of eight tags. Low battery power is signaled by an alarm sound from each tag. You may buy another set if you need more tags.

Persons with dementia sometimes remove the tags from the belongings because they forget why tags are attached to the belongings. In such a case, place the tag in a small bag (like a lucky charm), and attach a photo of the person's grandchild with a message saying "This is my present. Do not remove." and use chains so that the tags will not easily be removed. Similar products can be found online with keywords "finder" and "locater."

Related Topics —An experiment for finding items—

An experiment was conducted with a video recording system (Yasuda, Iwamoto, & Nakamura, 2003b). A CCD camera with a microphone was attached to the brim of a hat and it was connected to a digital video recorder on the waist of the user (Figure 4-3). The video camera was able to record what the user saw and heard (e.g., the faces and voices of people around them, and what the user touched or picked up). The participant of the experiment wore this system and was asked to hide five items in four rooms nearby. Then, an examiner tried to find the items without playing back the recording; only one item was found after 29 minutes of searching. Next, by searching for the

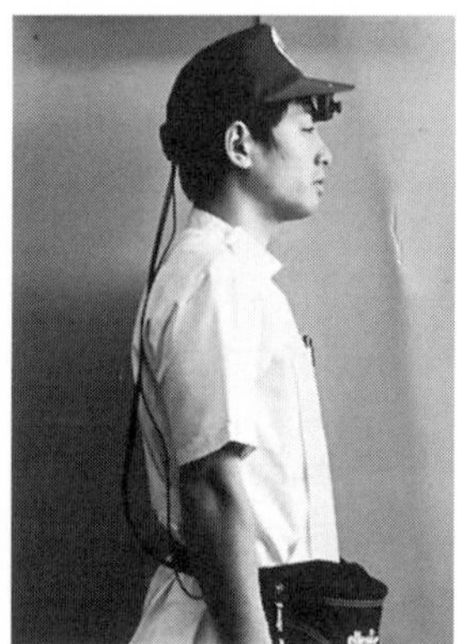

Figure 4-3 Video recording system

items while playing back the recording, it took only 8 minutes to find all of the remaining items.

Wireless tracking devices available today require the attachment of tags to the items before using them. Users who often forget the fact that they forget, however, tend to say this kind of device is "unnecessary." Currently, research is in progress to search for lost items by using videos and AI algorithms, without attaching the tags beforehand, regardless of whether users have the consciousness of forgetting or not.

Recently, there are small video devices that can record for 12 hours continuously. A portable camera *"Narrative Clip"* by Narrative takes one picture every 10 seconds to a minute. If you wear it for a day, you can capture almost all of the major events in your daily life. The photos are then uploaded to the Cloud and can be viewed remotely by family members. If you often forget, for example, locations of your belongings, you or your family can review the photos and organize your belongings at the end of the day. These are called life log cameras.

1.4 Devices to prevent forgetting belongings

Persons with MCI and dementia often forget to take important things with them when they leave the house. "*Doorganizer*" by Monkey Business is a device with small pockets that can be hung on a doorknob. "*Tower*" by Yamazaki has three big pockets with magnets in which plastic bags or magazines can be stored. Some persons are advised to tape a list of things to take out on the inside of the door and to check it before leaving the house. Separate lists can be made for different destinations (e.g., shopping, or hospital).

Some people tend to forget their belongings after putting them down. A device was developed to prevent people from leaving their bags behind. The main unit is attached to your clothes and a tag is attached to, for example, your bag or smartphone; the main unit emits an alarm sound when you are separated from your bag or smartphone. The device, "*Hanareruto Araamu* [alarm emits if you leave]" by Revex, will sound an alarm when you leave your tagged belonging, and it functions in the reverse way as well, to alarm when you get closer to the object. For instance, if you attach the main unit to the toilet at home and attach its tag to a person with dementia, the main unit will produce a sound when he/she approaches the toilet. If the main unit is attached to a family member and the tag is attached to the person, it will prevent him/her from getting separated from the family member, such as in a crowded market. The device, "*Hitokoko* [a person is here]" by Authentic Japan, has similar functions. It can be used in an underground mall, since it does not use GPS.

1.5 Timers

Kitchen timers, which are sold in dollar stores, are useful for remembering everyday tasks, if you forget what you ought to do over several minutes or hours (e.g., boiling water, doing laundry, and cooking). "*Double Timer*" by Dretec can set alarms for multiple tasks on the one device. Hang the timer around your neck to hear its alarm when you are moving about. If you cannot recall the tasks to do when the alarm sounds, create a memo-pad equipped with a timer, a pencil and scratch paper, and write down the tasks. After finishing one task, cross it off the list, and do the next task when the alarm sounds. This procedure will insure that all the daily tasks are done in order. The device, "*Oshirase* [message] *Timer COK-TT1*" by Ohm Electric, warns of the remaining time by sending a message such as "five minutes remaining." Smartphone timer apps are easy to use because you can set it up to say "Set the timer in seven minutes."

1.6 Device for voice guidance with human detecting sensor

Some persons with dementia keep on failing to do certain things properly in the same situation. For example, there are persons who fail to find the toilet, causing incontinence. Clinicians may recommend leaving the bathroom door open and the bathroom light on to facilitate finding the toilet in time. Using a voice-guided device is another option. This device installed in the bathroom will detect when someone is approaching and will produce a recorded voice message, "The toilet is here." Even though the device will warn any person who approaches the bathroom, it will not take long before family members get used to the voice and ignore it.

There was the case of a person who always left his cane in the bathroom. To deal with this problem, the instruction "Please take your cane when you leave" was recorded in the voice-guided device and it was set at the entrance of the bathroom to output the message as he approached the door. He stopped leaving his cane in the bathroom.

There was also the case of a person with dementia who used to get lost on the way to the bathroom in the middle of the night. The problem was resolved by placing the device at the door of his room. The recording told him "The bathroom is on your right" when he approached the door.

The device shown in Figure 4-4 is "*Onsei annaiki* [voice guidance] *Type S*" by Escor. The voice is relatively clear, and 15 voice guidance messages are pre-recorded so that you can choose the ones that are appropriate for the location. If you do not find a message you need, you can record your message to the device using a PC. You can also install made-to-order messages at extra charge when you purchase the device. You can record long instructions or the answers to persons' repetitive questions such as, "Your bankbook is kept in a safe place. You don't need to worry;" "Please do not buy goods not listed on your memo-note." (set at the entrance door); and "Your lunch is in the fridge" (set in front of the fridge). You can also attach a photo of the person the user trusts.

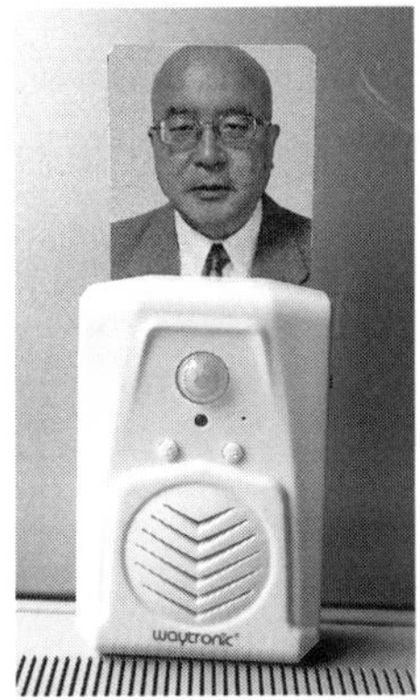

Figure 4-4 "*Onsei annaiki* [voice guidance] *Type S*"

1.7 Device with voice guidance and touch sensors

Some persons with dementia have to have catheters placed in their stomach, nose, urethra, etc. even after they are discharged from hospitals. Those who have dementia often forget why these catheters are inserted and try to pull them out, which makes round-the-clock surveillance by family members necessary. Escor and I made a prototype of a device that includes a string of touch sensors to manage this problem in 2007. A catheter will be wrapped by these sensors. Whenever a person with dementia touches the sensor-wrapped catheter, the device will play a recorded message telling him/her why the catheter is there and s/he should not pull it out (Figure 4-5). This system proved to be partially effective in reducing the number of pulling behaviors. I hope another company will commercialize such a device.

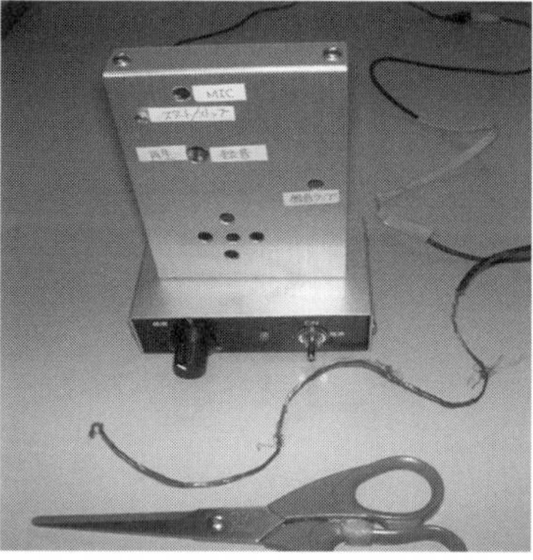

Figure 4-5 Device for voice guidance with touching sensor

1.8 Presenting information during the night

Some persons with dementia decide to "go home" or get restless in the night. It may be because when they wake up, they cannot recall where they are and why they are there. To provide information immediately after awakening, an electric memo-board, "*Black Board*" is useful. Written words on the board shine brightly. Turn on its light and place it where it can be seen immediately when they wake up. Write a message like "I am staying at my daughter's house." Whether the information is true or not does not matter, but it is important to write information that he/she will accept readily. The board can be hung in the corridor as a sign or directions to the bathroom (Figure 4-6).

There was an inpatient who tried to get over the bars of her bed to go to

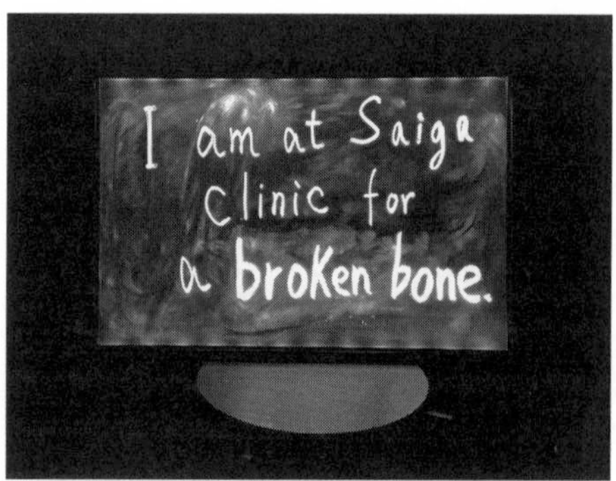

Figure 4-6 "*Black Board*"

the bathroom during the night, forgetting that she had broken her leg. The "*Black Board*" was hung from the ceiling above her feet so that she read the following message when she woke up, "If you need to use the bathroom, please press the call button." Then she stopped trying to get over the bars. A young female with a brain injury became restless during the night. Her family member wrote the message, "Dear ××, we will come and see you at ×× o'clock" and placed it where she could see it. Since then, she became calm. This board can be used at home, too.

1.9 Responding to repetitive questions

Voice-output communication aids (VOCA) are useful for people who ask the same repetitive questions. Figure 4-7 shows two examples of VOCA. For repetitive questions such as, "What's the date today?" and "When can I get my pension money?" record the respective answers onto separate buttons of the device and put a label on each. Pressing a button for the question, the person with dementia can listen to the answers anytime. The number of buttons is optional, and one of them can be worn on the users arm.

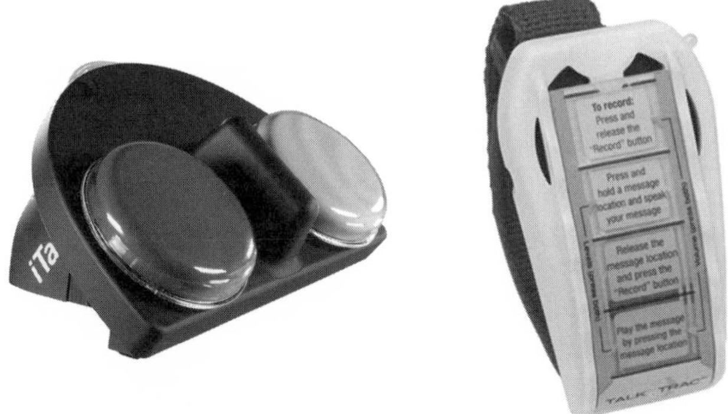

Figure 4-7 Voice-output communication aids
Source: Pacific Supply, https://www.p-supply.co.jp/.

1.10 Recalling an errand in the house

Recently, various shapes of keychain-type small recorders are sold for about 6–10 dollars. The round shape-type can be hung from the neck as a pendant, or attached to clothes with a pin on the back. We sometimes go somewhere in the house for an errand, but forget the purpose on the way.

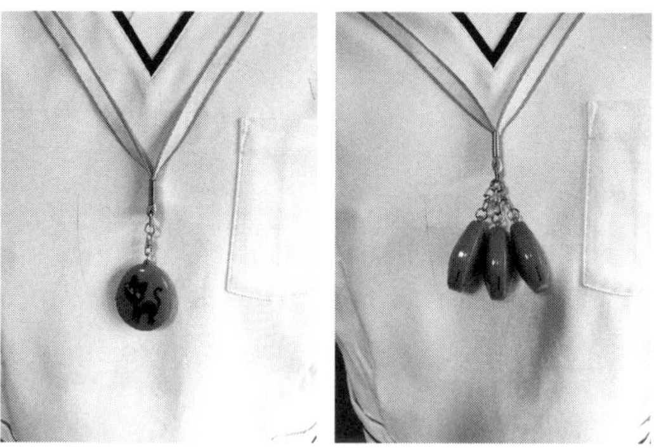

Figure 4-8 Small keychain-type recorders

We can make a recording on these devices before going and play it back if we forget. It is faster than taking a memo. The recording durations are 5–15 seconds. Similar to VOCA in the above section, this device can be used for persons who ask the same question repeatedly; the answer can be recorded by family members and played back by users when necessary. If users tend to ask several questions repeatedly in a day, several key holders can be used (Figure 4-8).

2. Videos, games, toys, dolls, and robots

2.1 Videos for severe dementia

When persons with severe dementia lose interest in conversations or watching TV dramas, family members may record TV programs of particular interest to that person, such as tennis, baseball games, and old music. Some persons with moderate dementia like TV programs for children. For example, Japanese TV programs such as *anime* movies for Japanese old tales are featured with gentle narration and beautiful pictures which even the healthy elderly like. Whenever the person is getting restless, the family member can show one of these programs promptly. These programs, however, may become difficult for them to enjoy when the dementia becomes more severe. There may be many old photos and videos on the Internet that persons with severe dementia might still enjoy. Photos and videos that have received good reactions so far from the persons are those of babies, smiling faces, cute animals, funny faces made by comedians, and scenes of fireworks.

Persons can simply enjoy the pleasant scenes without having to memorize contexts and the constantly changing scenes may make human beings react instinctively. In fact, some babies and adults become quiet in a car while they are looking at the moving scenery. One can find many videos of moving scenery over the Internet (views from car/train windows, drones, and planes, for example). Videos of people walking, running around the town, or hiking in the mountains are also useful.

Persons with moderate or severe dementia may suddenly become restless. Getting the person to watch a video can be difficult when they are moving around. It may be easier to get their attention if a tablet is hung from the professional caregiver's neck. This method can also be used to show the answers to repetitive questions after the verbal answers are changed into text via a verbal recognition application (see Hickey & Bourgeois (2018) and Astell et al. (2019) for other activities).

2.2 Games

A person with moderate frontotemporal dementia played the card game "Solitaire" on his PC for a few hours at a time. While he was playing the game in the mornings and evenings, his wife did the household chores. When he came to the Memory Clinic, he tried to leave the room immediately. To prevent him from wanting to leave, I scattered playing cards on the desk before he entered. While he concentrated on putting the cards in order, I was able to talk with his wife. Some persons with frontotemporal dementia are not interested in talking with other people; they seem more relaxed when they are concentrating on something interesting, such as a game. Therefore, card games and tablet game applications may help to keep them comfortable. As they also tend to perform the same tasks at the same times every day, it is important for family members to keep a consistent routine for their daily tasks.

2.3 Toys

Some persons with dementia show symptoms of restlessness, paranoia, and challenging problems. The causes are varied, but having something on which to concentrate may reduce the frequency of such behaviors. Redirection techniques can be used to prevent an expected behavior such as, "I want to go home." Today, we can buy traditional toys that the elderly used to play with in their childhood. Figure 4-9 is a "Memory box" (Bourgeois,

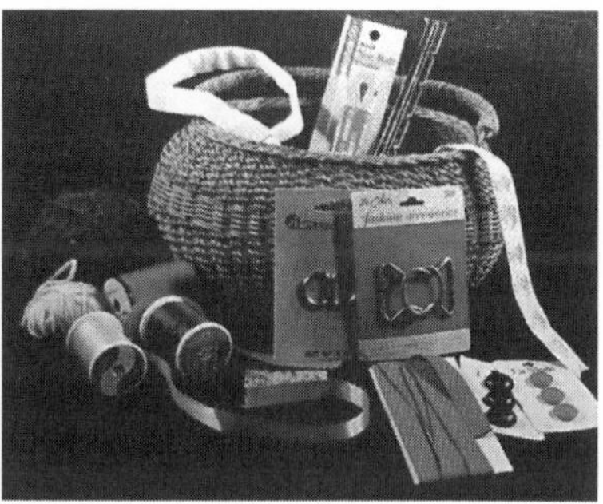

Figure 4-9 Memory box (sewing basket)
Source: Bourgeois (2014).

2014). I also created a memory box for Japanese elderly. It is a collection of old toys, dolls, and picture books that were safe and enjoyable. They served as prompts for sharing reminiscences with others. Some persons with severe dementia repeat the same movements. For such persons, you may be able to use a toy "*Mugen Putiputi* [infinite bubble wrap]" by Bandai that makes a pleasant sound when you press an elastic bubble with your fingers. Even healthy people enjoy it for a long time.

2.4 Dolls

Persons with dementia often love taking care of dolls. It appears that women like baby dolls and stuffed animals, while men prefer robot toys. Family members should have the person help to choose their own dolls or robots by observing their reactions to specific items in the shop. There are reports that persons who feel anxiety at night are able to sleep calmly with dolls. Takara Tomy's dolls "*Suyasuya* [sleep well] *melody series*" produce slow music and sounds similar to those heard in the womb. A huggable pillow, "Hugvi" by Veston, is effective with the IC Rec or a radio in a pocket on the pillow; some of them calm down with these sounds or music.

Various types of dolls are sold today. Some examples are: "*Oriko* [clever] *Kumatan*" by Fusion Marketing which will tell you fairy-tales; "*Special osewa* [take care] *set*" by Toysrus which is made for users to take care of by using baby bottles and nappies; "*Oshaberi* [speaking] *Maakun*" by Partners which will talk to you using short sentences and play word game; "*Popochan Onbu to dakko* [carrying baby on back]" by People which you can hug and play piggyback; and "*Unitan*" by Unicare which will announce the times for medicines and the toilet using the voices of family members. Few dolls,

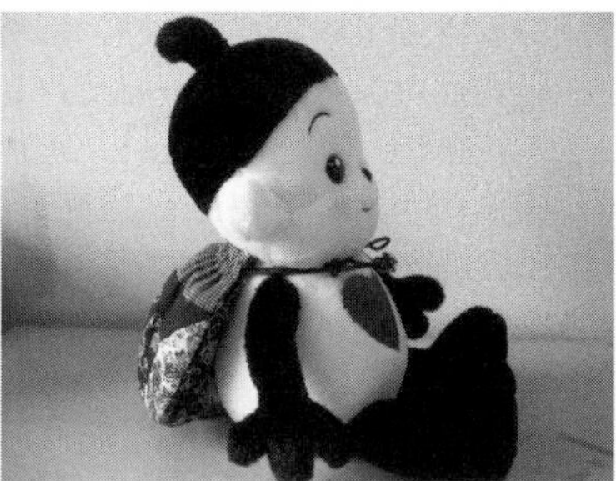

Figure 4-10 Doll with IC Recorder on its back

however, speak the way you might wish. As introduced in Chapter 3, you could record messages and songs into the Sony IC Recorder (ICD-PX240), put it in a cloth pocket, and sew the pocket onto the back of a doll. In this way, the personalized messages or songs can be played when they are desired (Figure 4-10). A button-type speaker, "*Pechat*" produced jointly by Hakuhodo, Ai-Studio and Monom, was attached to a stuffed doll. Family members choose the words and songs from the smartphone's application to be heard through the speaker. It also has a function for repeating words of users.

Related Topics —Persons who refuse to take a bath—

Some persons refuse to take a bath at home when their dementia deteriorates. Family members may try to use the IC Recorders, a waterproof doll, and/or music in order to persuade them to have a bath. It might be helpful to use a tablet computer to show videos of people taking an outdoor bath surrounded by beautiful scenery, with bath-related songs. When persons go to day-care centers, they should have a bath there since human resources and equipment are available for that purpose. If they refuse to take a bath there for the reason that they think the bath is not clean, you can arrange for them to have a bath before the other people take theirs. A husband persuaded his wife by saying, "Having a bath in the center is legalized for the members there." If persons suffer from incontinence, professional caregivers should arrange for them to put on a pair of disposable diapers right after having a bath in the center.

2.5 Stuffed toys

There are many kinds of stuffed toys in the shape of animals that talk available today. Following are some examples; "*Hello! Uu-nyan*" by Takara

Tomy (which will respond to you if you talk to them); "*Aiken* [pet dog] *Tetsu*" by Iwata (which will follow you); "*Oshaberi* [speaking] *Shibajiro*" by Iwaya (which will tell you the day and time); "*Walking talking babbie*" by Bestever Japan (which will walk if you talk to it); and "*Prin-chan*" by Osuto (which will perform various actions).

An animal-like doll, "*Maneshite Oshaberi* [echolalic speaking]" by Yamani, repeats words like a parrot. This doll also shakes its body when it detects TV sounds. Recently I loaned this doll to a person who was experiencing moderate visual hallucinations. The doll was helpful in reducing the number of hallucinations by diverting her attention and increasing her level of awareness to the doll. A doll called "*Hello! Zooma*" by Takara Tomy was loaned to another person. As this doll moves around freely, an electric cord was put around the doll's neck to limit its zone of movement (Figure 4-11). The care-manager for the person reported that the doll had the effect of attracting and maintaining her attention. It has been observed that persons with dementia calm down when they watch moving fish in an aquarium. The toy, "*Aquarium*," has fish-like toys swimming within it. Several types of tanks with artificial fish are on the market including one within a photo frame and a plastic bottle in which fish are swimming.

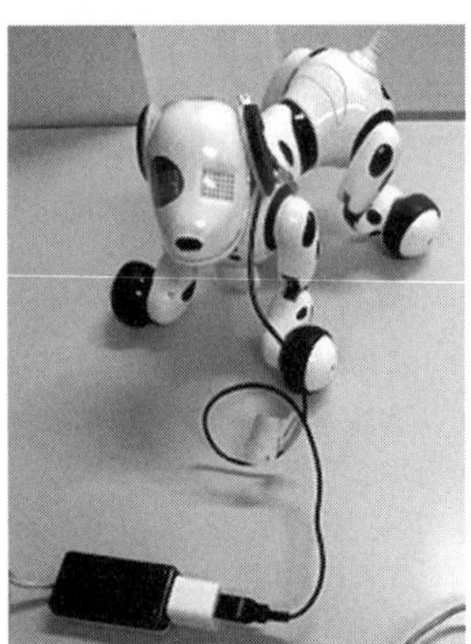

Figure 4-11 *Hello! Zooma* by Takara Tomy

Related Topics —Doll Phenomenon: Are dolls as lovable as people?—

Persons with severe dementia often love and take care of dolls as if they were alive. It is similar to the situation when they talk to faces on posters and newscasters on TV. Faces on posters and newscasters on TV are two-dimensional and virtual objects; but persons with dementia may think that these images are actual living and three-dimensional beings due to impairments of visual processing. Nevertheless, there are many reports of persons with dementia displaying positive, nurturing behaviors when taking care of dolls. This may be related to their memories of taking care of their own children. They may take care of dolls with a sense of charity over them, too. Doll therapy is based on such mentality of them (see Hickey & Bourgeois (2018) for related information).

2.6 Robots in the marketplace

An example of a talking baby robot for the elderly is "*Sumaibi S*" by New Life Frontier. "*BOCCO*" by Yukai Engineering is another robot-shaped toy with voice-recording function. "*XINGO*" by OPUS ONE is a robot speaker that can dance to music. It has more than 230 types of movement patterns. Users can compose different dances with these patterns using their app. "*Shabette* [speaking] *robo*" by NTT Docomo & NEC is a type of robot that talks through a smartphone. The robot, "*Telenoido*" by Telend Care, allows its user to communicate remotely with other people, and the facial expressions of this robot can be manipulated. With "*Tapia*" robot by MJI, you can observe users, have a conversation with and without videos, and play music for them. Robots with sensors tell family members via smartphone whether users are taking their medicines. "*Chapit*" by Ray Tron is a robot with which you can have a conversation, play games, and receive daily schedule information. In addition, it can control your home appliances. "*Robi jr.*" by Takara Tomy is a robot that can sing, output messages, and dance. You can talk with a robot called "*Robohon*" by Sharp; it enables people to have remote communication using its camera. "*Baku-sho* [laughing] *Taro*" by Takara Tomy is a robot with a radio-controlled clock, that tells jokes automatically at scheduled times, as well as manually.

A more expensive robot designed for care facilities is the "*NAO*" by Aldebaran Robotics. This robot can produce songs, ask questions, and respond to simple questions. "*PARO*" by Intelligent System is a seal-shaped robot that comforts users by responding vocally to their touch and voice. "*Pepper*" by Softbank is a programmable robot designed to interact with humans through speech recognition software. Application programs for the *Pepper* are actively being developed by many researchers.

Recently, several small and reasonably-priced AI robots have appeared on the market. "*COZMO*" by Takara Tomy will move towards a familiar person to engage with them by automatically recognizing people and objects. It is regrettable that we still have no robots dedicated to assist with the daily activities of persons with dementia. In the future, we expect that dementia-support robots will be developed and made available preferably on a rental basis to support their daily activities (see Section 2.9 in Chapter 7).

3. Safety and security devices

The installation of fire, smoke and gas alarm systems in places where persons with dementia reside is widely mandated in many countries. Stoves that use induction-heating (IH) or a type of sensor for boil-dry protection are increasing the safety of the kitchen. IH stovetops are provided for free to elderly citizens in some cities in Japan. For a gas-oven, it is desirable to choose the type that a user is familiar with, namely the turn type or push type ignition method. Same is true for a microwave; choose the one that the user finds easy to operate. Kerosine heaters are potentially high risk of causing fire. Electric candles and electric incense are recommended for the family altars in place of real ones. If one chooses to use real candles, short candles and fire-protection mats should be used.

Recently, there are automatic fire extinguishers for homes that sprinkle water or fire extinguishing powder when fire is detected. Several types are available such as a range hood type, wall-mounted type, and ceiling type; and installation of these devices does not require complicated remodifications. The city of Sapporo subsidizes their installation.

It is ideal to use a system that heats up and supplies/stops water automatically for the bath. An alarm "*Furoppii*" by takagi signals when the water reaches a certain level and when the water is heated to a certain temperature. When a water-proof speaker and a smartphone are connected, conversation is possible between family members outside and persons with dementia inside the bathroom, and the family members can give instructions such as, "put shampoo on your hair."

Water faucet control systems, such as "*Mizupita* [stop water]" by Idex, and "*Aqua-auto*" by Toto, prevent forgetting to turn off the water. Lighting equipment with sensors that detect human presence/absence and turn on and off automatically, prevents forgetting to turn off lights. Motion-detection equipment can be placed in front of, or inside, the bathroom to signal the location of the toilet, and it can be placed near steps or stairs to prevent falls. Recently, voice-operating light fixtures became available.

To prevent undesirable behaviors, such as persons with dementia pulling out electric cords of appliances from outlets, the "*Konsento* [plug] *cover*" can be used. Utility companies (e.g., Tepco) provide services for controlling gas lines. Air-conditioners can be controlled remotely using a smartphone to prevent heatstroke. In addition, a system called "*Smart appliances*" controls your appliances (e.g., refrigerator, washing machine, microwave, rice cooker) via the Internet. These are called the Internet of Things (IoT). If you connect a smart-plug and home appliances (lighting, electric fan, TV, etc.) to a smart speaker, you can start and stop these appliances by your voice. You can also operate them remotely.

Many home appliances have a switch button to be pressed with a finger. "*SwitchBot*" by SwitchBot can be attached to these switches so that one can operate them remotely (Figure 4-12). Bars of a SwitchBot rotate and press the switch of the device to which it is attached. It also has a timer function.

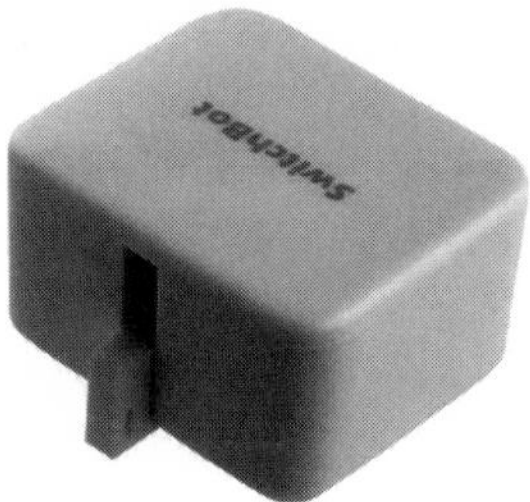

Figure 4-12 SwitchBot
Source: SwitchBot, https://sumahome.jp/archives/3428.

3.1 Various types of keys

Some people worry about whether they have locked the door of their house while they are away. A key case named "*Raku* [easy] *key case*" by Sankyoriken shows the time a user last took her/his key out from it, and a key, "*ChecKey*" by Miwa, changes the color of a part of the key every time it is used to lock the door. When your key is misplaced, a "*Keyholder-shape key-finder*" (produced by many companies) signals the location of the key by emitting sounds. Recently, there are many ways to open locks, including cards, PIN numbers, fingerprints, or smartphones. You may have to give a spare key to someone such as a visiting professional caregiver. In such a case, hang a small box called "*Key stock handy*" by Nomura Tech on the doorknob and put a spare key in it, and notify him/her of the box password.

To prevent persons with dementia from going out alone and getting lost, an inside lock, "*Hitoride dekakenaide* [do not leave alone]" by Guard Lock, can be installed on the door. To prevent them from opening the refrigerator, cabinets, and drawers, the "*Torenai-zo* [cannot remove]" by Hobby House Itou can be used. Although various locks are available in shops, using locks should be the last measure. It is better to first use "prevention" messages as **the strategy of presenting information in advance** by using devices such as the IC Recorder and devices for voice-guidance mentioned in Chapter 3.

3.2 Money and security boxes

Some people are worried that they have not received a monthly pension. Bourgeois (2014) created a pseudo letter from the bank, pasted the official identifying information onto a blank paper, and typed a new reassuring letter. When people ask about their banking situation, the family members can respond by showing this letter.

Some others feel anxious if they do not have cash with them. I recommend that they paste on the wall some bills in a clear hard-type file with a note saying "For Emergency". This file is called "*misegane* [showing money] *file*." This can lessen their obsession about cash because they can have some cash to use when necessary (Figure 4-13).

When dementia worsens, a person will not be able to use cash anymore. They should get used to using cards when they still can. Family members or guardians can set a limit to the usable amount in order to prevent excessive spending.

Some persons forget where they put their bankbook and may call the police, believing that someone, including their family members, has stolen

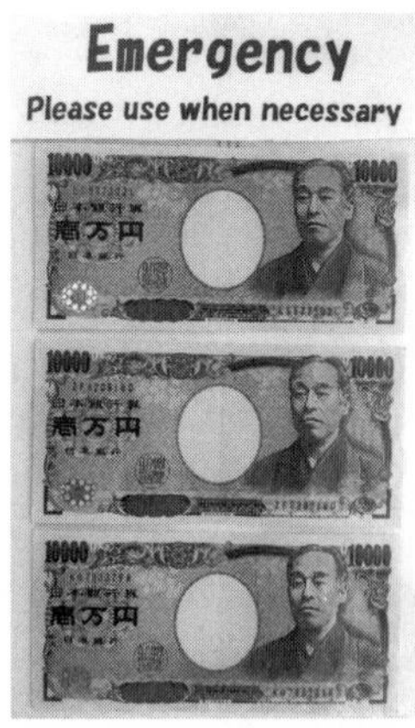

Figure 4-13 "*Misegane* [showing money] *file*"

it. This behavior is called "delusions of theft." Even if their room is locked, they may say that someone came into the room using a spare key. The typical advice to family members is to look for the "stolen" object together with them (redirection technique); an alternative method is to use one of the tracking devices for searching for objects described earlier in this chapter.

Today, you can buy a "security lock box" for a low price. Security boxes with fingerprint or biometric authentication are also available on the market for a few hundred dollars. There is a programmable timed lock box, "Time lock safety box," that can be opened at specific times such as when the family member is with the person. Keeping the person's bankbook and smartphone, as well as alcoholic drinks and cigarettes, in the safety box allows the family member to control the person's access to those things. Several transparent safety boxes are also available. If persons are worried because they cannot see the contents, this box may be better. Family members can install a motion-detection video recording device, such as "*Home security Daruma-shape camera*" by Amexα, and show the recording to them to confirm that no one opened his/her safety box. You can also use a safe-deposit box that banks lend to customers. Some local banks in Japan even have a service of withdrawing some money on your behalf from your savings up to a certain amount and delivering it to you.

3.3 Clocks and watches

The talking watch, "*Grus voice air wristwatch*," announces the time and date when buttons on the watch are pressed. The "*Himekuri* [daily] *voice air clock*" makes it easy to see the date and time. The clock, "*Voice clock Talk liner*" by Seiko, is suitable for persons with moderate dementia as it announces the time at fixed intervals. Some models can automatically play a recorded message at pre-set times. It is advisable to use these watches and clocks with a message board or a memory hanging pocket (see Chapters 2 and 5). When a person with dementia confuses the afternoon with morning, the pocket's IC Recorder can automatically play a recorded voice message such as, "It is ×× o'clock in the morning," or "It is ×× o'clock at night."

3.4 Supportive devices for hearing

Low-tech devices like a tin-can phone can be used as a hearing assistive device if nothing else is available at the moment. A person with hearing difficulty puts a capsule-shaped receiver on his/her ear, and a speaker puts another capsule on his mouth to speak. The two capsules are connected with a hose ("Oshaberi [speaking] hose" by Rakuten) or with an accordion-shaped pipe ("Moshi moshi [hello] phone" by Rakuten.) In my clinical experience, this simple device appears to be effective to some extent for persons with mild hearing difficulty, especially conversing at night.

A supportive device called "*Tele-amp III*" by Jiritsu Com, can amplify the volume of a telephone receiver. Persons with hearing difficulties often turn the volume up very high when they watch TV, which can annoy family members. A device called "*Mimimoto* [near your ears] *speaker*" (produced by various companies and a wireless type is also available) can improve the audibility of the TV without increasing the volume of the TV.

Hearing aids are available in many formats, including rechargeable, GPS-enabled, and smartphone-enabled. The volume of some hearing aids can be adjusted manually or digitally; others direct the audio from your smartphone (e.g., phone calls and GPS messages) directly into the hearing aid. Some people do not like to wear hearing aids because they may look older with the devices than they actually are. Unlike a pair of glasses, it takes time to get used to them. If you feel it necessary to wear them, you should go see an otologist and an audiologist. Hearing aids should be purchased at specialized shops. Today there are many types of hearing aids: a rental type, a type you can charge up by leaving it on the plate, a type you can locate easily with GPS, a type you can adjust the volume by remote control, and a type with which you can hear your smartphone directly and talk over the phone while the hearing aid is on. Sometimes persons misplace their hearing aids. To prevent this, create a routine of removing the hearing aids before bedtime or bathtime and placing them in a small box (or basket) that is kept in a designated place.

Simple sound amplifiers are available over the Internet. However, if a person with dementia refuses to wear hearing aids, family members can use a smartphone as a message board. There are apps with voice recognition features that can recognize verbal messages of family members, and convert them into written messages. Then the person can read the messages. This method is much quicker than writing down messages on the board.

3.5 Telephone and emergency contacts

There are telephone sets available on the market that are equipped with fraud prevention functions. Such telephones automatically record contents of a call, ask the caller's name, warn a user of a possible fraudulent or spam call, and alert a family member during such a call. Some can change your voice to a more masculine one. One telephone device called "*Otakkusu*" by Panasonic, can reject incoming calls not from the users' family members or friends.

With "*Hanaseru* [speak] *pendant Q-call*" by Kyuoki, users can make an emergency call by pushing a button. A telephone device called "*Smart-CARE*" by Iwatsu Manufacturing has a built-in microphone and a speaker, allowing a user to talk hands-free. It is equipped with a help button when a user needs some help, which subsequently lets the user talk to technical staff. "*Shilver-phon anshin* [safety phone for old people] *SVI*" by NTT contains a motion-detection sensor and if no movement of an elderly person has been detected for longer than an hour, it will report it to a family member or professional caregiver automatically. A system named "*Emergency call system*" by AI-Net, consists of a door phone, motion-detection sensors, an emergency contact feature, and a fire alarm feature; a user will receive periodic safety confirmation calls from the service company as well.

3.6 Room surveillance systems

Various surveillance systems for monitoring the elderly are available on the market. A surveillance system informs family members/professional caregivers when a user is operating their electric-pot, opening the refrigerator, using the bathroom, as well as detecting the user's general movements. Using a "*Mimamori Denchi* [surveillance battery]" is another easy way of surveillance. If you insert the battery into a remote controller such as a light, air-conditioner, or TV, their usage status will be notified to the family member's smartphone via the user's one. When they detect something unusual, they will call the user directly.

The system, "*Parumo mimamoriban* [surveillance]" by I-Seed, can control the temperature of the air conditioner remotely with a smartphone. A "network camera" device can observe the inside of a house and the movements of people within it. In many cases, the device operates with a combination of smartphones and cameras. Various companies sell this type of device today for approximately 100 dollars. The device, "*Mimamori* [surveillance] *TV phone Parumo*" by I-Seed, has multiple functions including ones to turn the direction of the camera, to have a videophone conversation, to take photos in the darkness, and to record the inside of the room. An example of a useful recording is one by which family members know when the user went out and what clothes they wore.

Motion-detection sensors for dangers around the beds of persons with dementia are available from companies such as Technos Group. Various sensor systems are sold for detecting risks when persons get up from their bed, grab the bars of the bed, put their legs on the floor mat, and so forth. These sensors can be purchased from hardware stores and internet websites. Some surveillance services are provided by municipal governments for free. Consult the administration of your city, care managers, local comprehensive support centers, and welfare-goods shops for available systems. Companies such as Secom, Fujitsu, and *Yasashiite* manage surveillance services using sensors and the Internet for approximately 10 dollars per month. As for the ethical issues of surveillance, see Astell et al. (2019) and Jotterand et al. (2019).

3.7 Prevention of going out alone

There are many tracking systems that notify family members when persons with dementia exit outside of their room or the house. The systems operate using sensors to detect their approach to the door. Some devices respond only to specified people and record automatically. Information about these systems can be found on the Internet using keywords such as, "detection for going out," "notification about wandering around," "transmitting device on doors/windows," "human detection," "wireless," "chimes," etc. The cost of these systems is approximately several hundred dollars.

A sensor-switch, "*Beruf infrared-ray sensor switch*" by Ichinen MTM, can turn on the TV and lights, and it can output a recoded voice message automatically. For example, at the entrance door a message can inform persons with dementia to not exit through the door.

3.8 Detecting locations

If persons with dementia have a smartphone, or a GPS tag, their location can be found. There are paid services whereby the staff members of security firms locate the persons and rush to them when they are lost. Secom leases the device, "*Kokosecom*," for approximately 9 dollars per month (for a standard type). There are also shoes installed with a GPS tag, "*Mimamoru* [surveillance] *shoes*" by Yume Yume Life. The detection device, "*Parumo docchi kun* [where abouts]" by I-Speed, can be attached to objects other than shoes, and it notifies family members of the person's location by detecting the vibrations when the person starts moving. It is installed with an

"*Area alert*" which sends emails to family members when they go out of the specified safety zone, and with a "*Timer alert*" which signals the location of persons at scheduled times. These can be rented for approximately 20 dollars per month.

Persons with dementia need to become accustomed to wearing the devices as soon as they get up in the morning. For this purpose, the IC Recorder or an alarm can notify them every morning to put on the device. It is also important to put the tag in a small bag or in the pocket inside of their clothes so that the devices will not be removed easily while they are wearing them. Or, the device can be attached to the instep of their shoe. Detection devices such as "*San flower mimamori* [surveillance] *service*" by Kato-Denki use no GPS. These devices are supposed to detect users inside of buildings as well as underground. Although locating the person using these devices and bringing them back home are possible, the best solution is to prevent them from going out by giving them the necessary messages in advance, as described in Chapter 3.

3.9 Incontinence

Advice relating to problems of incontinence can be obtained from "*Haisetu no komarigoto 110* [problems with toileting]" (Continence Action Society), and information about continence-related products is found at "*Mutsukian* [diapers house]." When a person with dementia begins having accidents, cover the floor and the walls with waterproof sheets as early as possible. When they urinate in a particular corner of a house, put training pads/sheets for pets on the floor. Placing something (e.g., a statue or poster) the person recognizes as valuable/holy there might also be effective.

Continence-related goods for persons in care facilities include "*Oshikko* [urine] *sensor*" by Tokuso (it vibrates when a diaper becomes wet) and "*Haisetsu* [excretion] *wearable DFree*" by Triple Japan (it estimates the amount of urine in the bladder and signals the timing to go to the bathroom via smartphone). An excretion detection system "*Aiserv*" by Shinto Kogyo is a system that detects the odor of feces and flatulence with a sensor inside the diaper and notifies it to the smartphone. The history of excretion can also be displayed, making it easy to predict. Since the professional caregiver does not open the diaper and wake up the wearer, the detection would be especially effective during the night.

The self-flushing toilet, "*Remote-control self-cleaning handle Nagaserumon* [can flush]" by Lixil is recommended for people who often forget

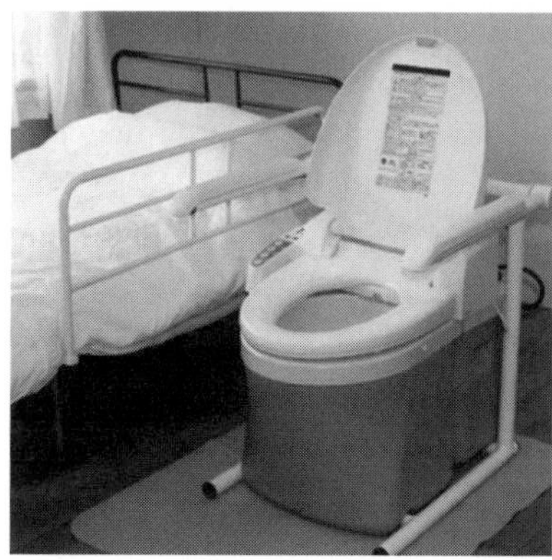

Figure 4-14 *Nagaseru poota kun* by AM
Note: Water-flushable bedside toilets.
Source: AM, http://www.pota-kun.jp/img/pamp.pdf.

to flush. This device is available for under 100 dollars. The "*Sojiguchi tsuki* [with cleaning hole] *public compact benki* [toilet]" by Toto is a type of toilet from which you can easily remove diapers when they are stuck in the toilet bowl. "*Nagaseru* [can flush] *poota kun*" by AM are water-flushable bedside toilets. The waste materials in the toilet basin are flushed by connecting its pipe to the lavatory pipes through the narrow opening of the windows (Figure 4-14). Recently, water-flushable and portable toilets with hand rails are on the market which can be used outside.

There are suction-operated urine collector systems such as, "*Skatto clean*" (with a urine receiving holder) by Paramount Bed. The "*Humany*" by Unicharm is a system in which a nappy pad is installed with a sensor, and when the sensor detects urine, it vacuums it up automatically.

An example of a product that vacuums, cleans, and disposes of waste materials automatically is "*Mainretto sawayaka* [fresh]" by NWIC (Figure 4-15). These systems are approved for purchase or rental using the Long-Term Care Insurance of Japan. Recently, I came up with an idea for a diaper cleaning system. The system would allow for vacuuming of waste, cleaning and drying of body parts while the user is wearing the diaper (search my website with "Kiyoshi Yasuda homepage"). These systems will help family members reduce their own burden of changing the user's diapers.

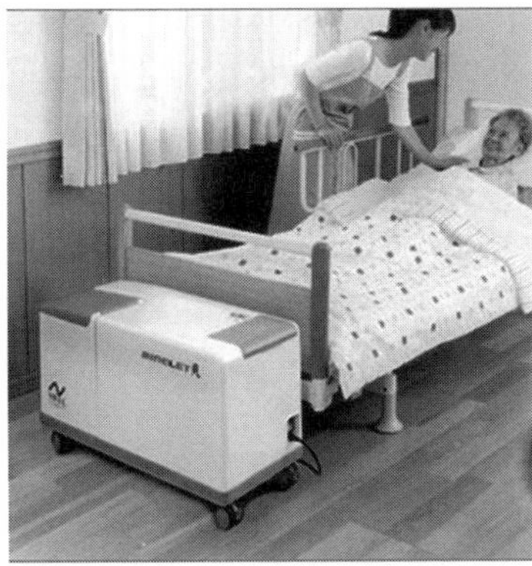

Figure 4-15 "*Mainretto sawayaka*"

Note: A product that vacuums, cleans, and disposes of waste materials.
Source: IID, https://www.rbbtoday.com/article/2013/01/06/100634.html.

4. Recently commercialized Middle-Tech ATs

4.1 Smart speaker and smart display

A smart speaker is a voice command device. It can be placed on the table for home usage. The device plays music, sets alarms, turns on and off the videophone and air conditioner, and manages a schedule through vocal commands. When asked general questions such as today's weather, News, or the meaning of words, the device will give you an answer if the questions are not too complex. You can have short chats with it, too. Smart speakers are sold for approximately 100–200 dollars, such as "*Google Home*" by Google. Sony's "*Xperia Hello!*" is rather expensive, but it enables the users to send/receive LINE messages, to talk on a videophone, to receive event schedules automatically, and to watch interiors by a rotating camera controlled remotely. A small smart speaker "*Google Home Mini*" by Google is also on the market.

Smart displays (smart speakers with a monitor) such as "*Echo Show*" by Amazon and "*Smart Display*" by Google are now available. As images and videos are shown on the monitor, such devices become more helpful for persons with dementia who often fail to recognize the visual images of faces, objects, and scenes as these are described verbally. Reminiscence therapy using photos can be conducted with this device.

Smart speakers and smart displays can control some electronic appliances by voice, and thus are very useful for persons with dementia when they gradually find it difficult to use those appliances. If they have difficulty learning how to manipulate the devices, write the instructions for using them on a card and attach it to the device.

4.2 Virtual reality

In the near future, VR (virtual reality) will become an effective Middle-Tech AT for persons with dementia. They may enjoy watching various videos within their full visual field if their eyes are covered with a goggle-like box. When their stage of dementia progresses, they may fail to scan their visual field and their eyes may lose focus. Wearing VR goggles, however, enables them to watch the moving images. A model of the goggles using a smartphone inserted into a cardboard box is also available for a low price. More video contents for this device should become available for elderly people in the future.

There are many persons with dementia who cannot accept or learn current events, such as the death of a relative. There was a person with severe dementia who was unable to remember her mother's death even after several years passed. When her daughter mentioned it, she accused her daughter saying, "That is not true. Did you kill her?" One of the coping methods would be to make a VR video in which the deceased mother explains what happened. The video of the mother can be created using her photo by moving the mouth in coordination with artificial utterance (Nakatani, Saiki, Nakamura et al., 2018). Today, some VR systems can even present smells and vibration (see D'Cunha, Nguyen, Naumovski et al. (2019) for other information).

4.3 Smartwatch

The watch-shaped information device, smartwatch, enables us to look at emails without taking the smartphone out of the pocket. It also has convenient functions such as a calculator, mobile wallet, and unlocking your door remotely with your smartphone. It is equipped with sensors to check the health conditions of a user such as pulse rate, step counting, sweat volume, skin temperature, respiratory rate, blood pressure, blood oxygen level, electrocardiographic monitor, stress level and sleep status (sleep time, quality, snoring, breathing). Recent versions of the watch have more functions such as a GPS, an acceleration sensor, a microphone for recording, and a speaker and many music files.

When these functions are utilized, the users' current behaviors such as eating, exercising, going shopping, and listening to audio messages will be recognized based on arm movements, GPS tracking, and speech monitoring. Automatic instructions for taking medicines after meals, confirming shopping lists, and recording messages may be given to users, as well as providing them with health advice. The smartwatch will definitely become a helpful AT for healthy elderly and persons with MCI.

4.4 Smart pendant

Users usually take the wrist-watch off when they are home or wash their hands. Accordingly, automatic instructions would be difficult to be given to users in their homes. Therefore, I created a smart pendant by modifying the

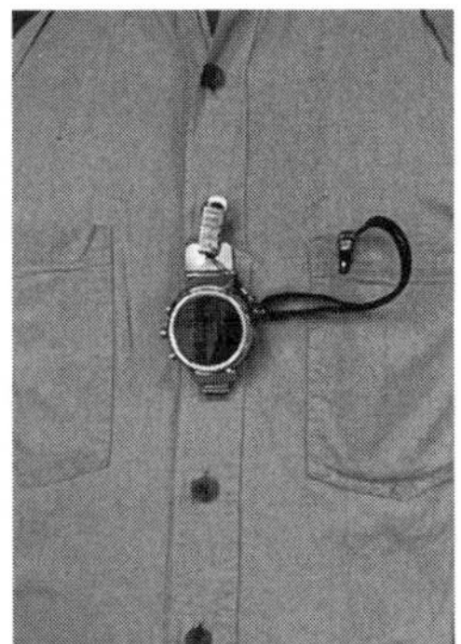
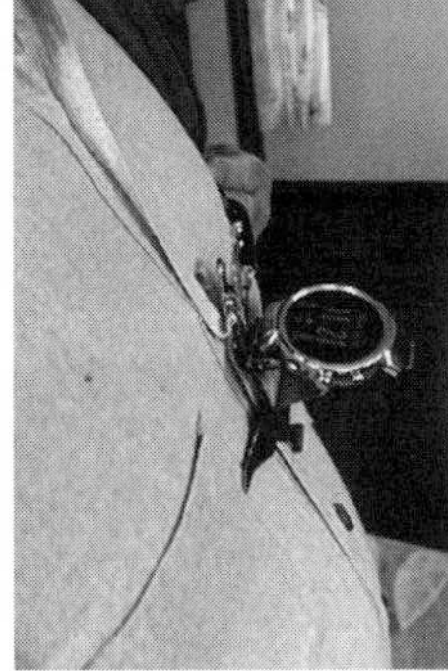

Figure 4-16 "*Smart pendant*"
Note: The screen can lift to 90 degrees vertically.

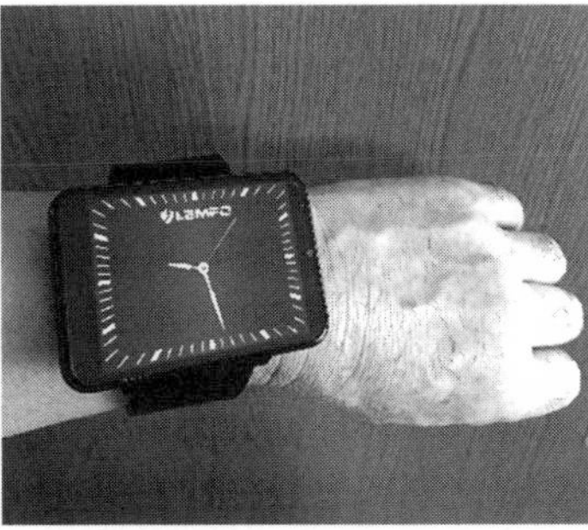

Figure 4-17 Smartwatch by Lemfo

smartwatch so that it will hang down from the neck or attached to clothes. By this modification, they can lift the screen up to 90 degrees vertically toward their face (Figure 4-16). They can look at the screen easily without raising their hands. This pendant will become a user-friendly wearable device if smartwatches with a big screen are used. "*CWAT219141H LEMT 3+32G*" by Lemfo has such a big square screen (about 7 × 5 cm) (Figure 4-17).

5. Sources of AT products

The National Rehabilitation Center for Peoples with Disabilities in Tokorozawa has the "Exhibition pavilion for welfare (supportive) devices for persons with dementia," with displays of local and international ATs. An appointment is needed to visit the pavilion (http://www.rehab.go.jp/ri/kaihatsu/dementia/modelj.html).

Some shops on the Internet in Japan have begun introducing and selling goods for caring for elderly people and for persons with dementia. Escor sells products such as guidebooks, DVDs, dolls, diaries, calendars for medicines, and a device for voice guidance with human detecting sensor. (https://escor.co.jp).

Other related online shops are as follows;

- "dfshop" sells and introduces items to help persons with dementia, or disabilities. (https://dfshop.thebase.in/)
- "CARETOWN" sells nursing care products. (http://caretown.info/)
- "E-SUPPLY" sells useful goods for the elderly and people with disabilities. (https://www.esupply.co.jp/senior/)

The products for persons with physical impairments are supplied to some extent on these Japanese websites. As introduced in this chapter, many supportive products related to MCI/dementia are also sold on the market. However, the number of such products available on these websites is extremely small compared to those in other countries.

- "A website for categorized ATs for the healthy elderly and MCI/dementia": I have collected about 250 possible ATs' data for persons with MCI/dementia. They were assigned to each of the 10 symptoms of MCI/dementia. In February 2022, the above categorized ATs were published on the following website. Customers can purchase them from the attached URL (https://monowasure.site/goods/).

An internet website in the U.S.A., "The Alzheimer's Store" sells various types of AT goods for persons with dementia (http://www.alzstore.com/shop-alzheimers-store-s/2054.htm). The goods are categorized into 20 groups, including clocks, music, dolls, incontinence, etc. They sell products such as a music and memories photo frame for reminiscence therapy, big posters to put on the doors to prevent persons with dementia from exiting, etc. There are some goods that are not available in Japan. For example, they sell a"Lock box"which comes with many tools (e.g., keys and screws) and drawers. As persons with severe dementia enjoy touching and feeling things, these products provide many opportunities for manipulating different types of objects.

Similar websites are as follows;

- "AlzProducts.co.uk" (https://www.alzproducts.co.uk)
- "Dementia shop Australia" (https://dementiashop.com.au/)
- "Alzheimer's Society: Online shop" (https://www.alzheimers.org.uk/)
- "Dementia aids and Equipment for care home" (https://www.careshop.co.uk/dementia-care)
- "Best Alzheimer's Product Store" (https://best-alzheimers-products.com/)
- "Artist life station: Best Alzheimer's Products (https://best-alzheimers-products.com/product/artist-life-station)
- "Alzheimer's Society Shop" (https://shop.alzheimers.org.uk/)
- "MindCare" (https://www.mindcarestore.com/)
- "dementiacareproducts" (https://www.dementiacareproducts.co.uk/reminiscence-products)
- "Lifted" (https://www.liftedcare.com/product-category/music-players/)

Related Topics —A working group for assisting inpatients—

At Chiba Rosai Hospital, a working group, the "Dementia Support Team," was established in 2009 to propose supportive measures for inpatients with dementia. The proposals included: when the inpatient was admitted to the hospital, asking the family member to bring an electric clock, photos, DVDs, and favorite items such as dolls, decorating their room in the old Japanese style, preparing a "Memory box" (Chapter 4) and a "Black Board" (Chapter 4), asking conversation volunteer companions to visit the inpatient for conversation, setting up the tablet and Wi-Fi systems so that they can have videophone conversations with family members (Chapter 6), and making video messages by using digital photo-frames (Chapter 6). It was also suggested that they use a nurse-call system that shows faces of inpatients and nurses, an alert system to signal when they leave the bed, "*Information terminal for the bedside*" by Vitas, a system to help hospital staff locate them in the hospital, and a low-floor bed "*Pettanko* [on the floor] *beds*" by Sanyo.

5.1 Summary of Chapter 4

Recently, the number of family members who utilize ATs is increasing. Hironobu Kudo is introducing effective tools for his mother's remote care (his mother is living alone and has moderate dementia) such as surveillance cameras for confirming her safety behaviors, smart speaker for automatic (repeated) verbal messages for her daily schedules, smart remote controller for starting of her favorite TV programs, SwitchBot for starting of appliances by pushing buttons remotely etc. See details on his website (https://40kaigo.net/).

Usability of the ATs introduced in this chapter varies depending on the situations and abilities of each user. Not all the devices introduced here have been tested by myself. Furthermore, since the time when this book was published, newer ATs have appeared on the market, some of them have been modified in their specifications, and some of them may have been discontinued. Contact the manufacturers for more information. Also, check the reputation and evaluations of each product on the Internet, or look for alternative devices.

More devices which could be used as AT will be produced in the future. What we need to do is not to think of how we can apply the devices after we get them, but rather to think in advance that if a device with certain functions is released, it can be adopted and solve a problem that the present AT cannot. Unless we always think of this kind of simulation, we will not be able to utilize newly developed devices as AT. If you are interested in new devices and systems, you should participate in engineer-related research groups or academic societies. If you register your name on the mailing list of the Japanese Society for Artificial Intelligence (https://www.ai-gakkai.or.jp/) or on those of related associations, you will receive emails about information related to academic conferences and professional workshops.

CHAPTER FIVE

Daily support using smartphones, clothing and others

1. Smartphones

Yasuda (2007a) recommended that the elderly and persons with MCI should make the most of cellphones. This is because they would get unprecedented support in many ways by using cellphones. Now, the cellphones have been replaced by smartphones. Application programs (app) that recent smartphones provide by default include maps, calendars, clocks, pedometers, cameras, weather forecasts, transportation guidance, and so on.

Now, some of the apps can be activated by just talking to your smartphone, such as: “OK google, make a call to ××,” “OK google, set an alarm for after 20 minutes,” etc. The accuracy of recognizing verbal commands is improved when environmental noise is limited, and your pronunciation is clear. Furthermore, if you put your schedule in the smartphone in advance, it will respond to a query relating to your personal schedule, e.g., “What is my schedule for today?” The map app can show a route between your present location and the destination on a regional map if you ask, “How do I get to the hospital from here?”

The smartphone may be an “electronic secretary” for elderly people if they make good use of it. An elderly user who had early-onset dementia called it a “magic tool.” It takes many months, however, to become accustomed to the smartphone, and therefore, the elderly should begin using it as their Middle-Tech AT as early as possible. The family members should learn first how to use it so that they can teach it to the persons with MCI and mild dementia.

Some smartphones, such as Docomo’s “*rakuraku* [too easy] *phone*,” are designed for elderly users. Their interfaces are relatively easy to use and the screens are wide so that inputting operations manually is reasonably easy. On the other hand, the interfaces of smartphones for ordinary people can be altered for the elderly by installing apps such as "*Kantan* [simple] *home*" by KDDI. Softbank's "*Simple Smartphone*" provides a service called "*Assist Smartphone*" for users with disabilities. With this service family members can set up and manage the schedules of the users on their smartphones using the family members' devices. The family members also can watch over the users' behaviors with their smartphones. A similar remote-control app called "*TeamViewer*" by Team viewer can help the users learn remotely how to use their smartphones.

Smartphones developed for children's use are simple, light, and sold at reasonable prices. This type has special functions that family members may find useful, including the one that signals when users leave home. They can set the limit of number of calls and destinations that users can make to prevent excessive charges on the phone bill. In addition, if they show the particular icons of familiar persons on their own screens all the time, they can call a specific person quickly. For example, if their husband with dementia gets angry suddenly, she can ring her daughter and then the daughter may call back immediately. She may calm her father. The Apple "iPhone" does not have any specific versions for the elderly or for children. Therefore, the smartphones and apps referred to in the following sections are for the Android. Similar apps are also available for iPhones. The apps described are free for use in many cases.

1.1 Surveillance and communication

"*Sumakuro*" by System Friend is a stuffed doll with a smartphone inside, and it can receive and send short videos easily in order to watch over the elderly and to promote communication with remote families. When the elderly receive a video from the family members, the elderly can watch it simply by pressing a button, and their verbal responses and images will be immediately and automatically sent to the family members. A surveillance device called "*Picot*" by E&I is a box with a built-in smartphone. Without the Internet, you can automatically send photos and five-second voice messages at fixed times. The device is also equipped with a button to press after you take your medicines. The "*Mago* [grandchild] *channel*" by Chikaku enables you to see images sent to your smartphone enlarged on your TV monitor. "*Mimamori* [surveillance] *GPS app*" by Softbank is one of the many apps available for watching over the elderly.

1.2 Medicine-taking and schedule management

Using the apps for medications, such as "*Okusuri* [medicines] *note*" by Karada Note, you can set alarm signals for the times to take medications, such as between meals or before-and after-meals, and you can also record whether you have taken your medicines or not. These apps have the capability to send your family a message by pressing a button every time after you take your medicines. Other "*Schedule*" apps can also manage your daily schedules including medicine taking. A daily support app called "*Arata* [new]" by Insight was developed for persons with executive function disorder and memory impairments. Alarms and voice messages are outputted from their smartphones to let users know when to take medicines and other daily activities. The task to be done at present is always shown on the screen as well as the tasks to follow. This paid app is easy to use but it cannot be installed in some types of smartphone.

You can input your daily routine tasks into your smartphone by speaking, if you install the app "*Any.do*" by Any.Do in your device. A product called "*Tegaki* [handwritten] *memo alarm*" converts a handwritten memo to a reminder that will be presented later at a pre-set time. The app "*Remember the Milk*" by Remember the Milk is to prevent you from forgetting items to buy. In Chapter 3, many examples were introduced to assist you by using the "**alarm play-back**" of the Sony IC Recorder (ICD-PX240). An app similar to the function of the IC Recorder, "*Talking alarm*" by Mirolunapp is available today, although it requires that you press its stop button to discontinue the alarm sounds. You could use your old cell/smartphone, which you will not use as a phone, as your alarm device, if you leave it plugged into an outlet.

1.3 Health management

Currently, there are many apps that record daily exercises and activities to improve your health. "*Daily Workouts*" by Daily Workouts Apps LLC lets you exercise while watching a trainer's video on your smartphone. There are apps that encourage you to fall asleep with soothing music, and "*Sleep Cycle*" by Sleep Cycle AB analyzes your sleep patterns and wakes you up at an optimal time. Some apps will suggest a user to go to a hospital when she/he exhibits certain symptoms. "*COCOLOLO*" by WIN frontier can check your stress level after you place your fingers on the camera. If a user has a smartphone and a smartwatch, "*Hachi*" by AP TECH automatically sends biometric information such as heart rate and step numbers to a distant family member. An SOS function is also installed.

1.4 Recording conversations and speech recognition

It is recommended that the elderly record conversations and replay them to check the contents later. Persons with memory impairments are advised to do this especially when they receive long messages. An app called "*Voice Recorder*" by Splend APS is simple to use for recording conversations and the recorded items are listed chronologically. Additionally, a timer function is equipped to start recording automatically. For example, if you set the timer for your doctor's appointment, it will record the appointment and prevent you from forgetting the doctor's instructions. Some apps can transcribe the recorded speech into written text. If users send the transcription to their PC, they can save the messages to a diary file. An app for diary writing called "*Imagoto* [my day today]" by Aibri shows the events/messages of the day before, a week ago, three months ago, and a year ago. You can also create a book based on your diary entries at your own charge. The maximum of 500 pages can be included in the book with the explanation of each photo. You can choose your favorite cover from the choices given.

1.5 Browsing names and faces

The ability to recall persons' names and faces deteriorates as people get older. You can categorize the names in the address book on your smartphone into groups, such as family, colleagues, friends with the same interests, etc. Category names are easier to recall than each person's name. When you cannot recall the name of a person in front of you, for example, you can check the name by opening the address book while you are pretending as if a call came in. There is such a training for remembering people's names, but the better choice is to learn the compensatory method of using a smartphone as mentioned above. You may remember people's names but sometimes you are unable to recall their faces. You may ask the person if you can take a photo of their face when you meet them for the first time. With an app "*Skitch*" by Evernote, you can write the names on the photos.

You can learn people's names and faces by looking at them every day. I had a person with mild dementia who was reviewing relatives' faces in his smartphone's photos every night. The program "*everyStory*" by David Keene is an app with which you can attach a voice to the photos. If you feel it troublesome to put names on photos later on, you can take photos of people's faces and their business cards together when you meet them for the first time. Or you can ask them to introduce themselves while you are recording a video on your smartphone. This will help you remember their name, voice, facial expressions, and specific interactions.

1.6 Searching for belongings, cars, and other objects

The elderly often look for their wallet, a pair of glasses, or other items. This happens when they do not pay attention to where they put them. It becomes a serious problem when they forget where they placed their bankbooks and credit cards. To solve this problem, they can take photos of the items where they put them so that they can find them later. With an app "*Snapy*" by Schiz Tech, you can take photos quickly because a shutter button always appears on the top screen. The date of taking the photo is automatically added as well.

In Chapter 4, many devices for searching for belongings were described. There are smartphone apps, such as Bluetooth, and tags to help you find belongings. They let you know where belongings are by means of emitting sounds from the tags; however, the volume of the emitted sounds may be low for elderly people. Each tag is about the size of a big coin, and costs from 10 dollars to 20 dollars. You can connect and manage up to 10 tags with apps on your smartphone. If you lose the smartphone, you can find it by using the tags, although the usage of this function depends on the app.

A similar type of device called "*Mamorio*" by Mamorio helps you find your belongings by attaching a small tag to your bag or item. With this device, if you begin to move without taking your bag, for example, the device will notify you of the bag on your smartphone. Even after you walked far away, you can also find where you lost your bag on the map app. That is, if someone who happens to walk near the bag and has the same app on his/her smartphone, his/her smartphone automatically activates mobile relay transmission and notifies the location to your smartphone.

The "*Metal detector*" by Alexander Balyberdin is an app to help you find metal tools left behind in the grass or on the ground for activities such as farming, or gardening. You may forget where you parked your car in a large parking lot. In such a situation, you can use an app called "*Chushaichi* [parking place] *navi*." On the Internet you can find the rankings for these navigation systems for your parked car. Smarter systems are in the process of development whereby if your smartphone and car are parted, the location of your car will be registered automatically on your smartphone.

1.7 Location and direction (GPS apps)

If you need guidance traveling from one location to another, "*Google speech recognition*" software can guide you with verbal and written messages. If you get lost, the "*assist nabi*" by Softbank will show you the correct direction if you hold your smartphone forward. Another app, "*Google keep*," can be set to recognize when you get close to the supermarket, and then automatically show your shopping list.

Persons with Alzheimer's disease are likely to suffer from topographical disorientation. Thus, it is ideal for them to get used to a GPS app for route navigation. A person with early-onset dementia started cycling after he stopped driving a car. Although he sometimes lost his way, he succeeded in getting home by using the route navigation. "*Nabi Reco Lite*" by Amedia was developed for persons with visual impairment. Volunteers prepare the necessary route guidance in advance. Persons with dementia may be assisted by vibrations and voices of this app if their routes are fixed. When the severity of dementia progresses, they cannot maintain their independence by walking to their destination. In such cases, if the person has a smartphone with GPS or a small device with GPS, family members can find their location by using their smartphones (see Astell et al. (2019) for related information).

1.8 Group video conversation

Smartphone users are able to have a face-to-face conversation by using videophone apps such as Skype, LINE, Zoom, Facetime, and others. By watching users' faces and conversing, family members may check their physical and mental status, as well as their medication compliance. Recently, it became possible to organize conversational meetings with more than 10 people using Zoom, Skype and other platforms. The organization of peer-groups and family members' groups has become extremely easy. This is a breakthrough technology for assisting persons with disabilities and their family members. For example, a remote consultation "Pub" meeting can be held where participants discuss how to cope with various problems while drinking and eating in front of their smartphone or PC (see Section 2.4

in Chapter 8).

1.9 Supports by remote groups and Memory Sharing

It is becoming possible to support the daily life of a person with dementia by a remote group. For example, a remote support group could be set up using LINE. Persons with dementia can send messages on what they have done, what they have talked about, what they want to ask, and so forth to the group. The voice input function will probably be faster than using "finger-input" for the elderly if they speak clearly. If users take photos of the location of their personal items and upload the photos to the LINE group with a title for each photo, later they can find the items by the title. But if they still cannot find them, they can ask the other members with good memory in the support group for assistance. I would like to call this system as **Memory Sharing**.

Another helpful strategy would be for the support group members, for example, to take a video of how to use a microwave oven and upload it to the LINE program with the title "microwave oven." When users forget how to use the microwave oven, they can search the program with the term "microwave oven." They may be able to operate the oven while referring to the video on the LINE. If they still are having difficulty using the oven, they can ask group members for assistance by using their smartphone to show the oven and then their supporters can teach them how to use it in real time. If persons with dementia can get these remote supports, they can reduce the number of questions they ask family members. This support can be described as the remote utilization of the younger person's surplus memory for the elderly. It would be even better if a reward system could be created in which young people are given something, such as volunteer coupons, every time they help the elderly. The **Memory Sharing** system should be implemented more widely from now on.

Users can immediately use the LINE app by pressing a button on the smartphone screen. The LINE always notifies its users about newly arrived information by showing the number of messages not checked beside the icon on the screen. LINE will be an important app for remote support (Figure 5-1). With "*ANYTIMS*" by ANYTIMS, you can easily ask for help with errands such as house cleaning or walking your pet to registered supporters who have the same app and live nearby.

The transceiver system "*BONX Grip*" by BONX can be used by up to 10 people at the same time by downloading the app to their smartphones and

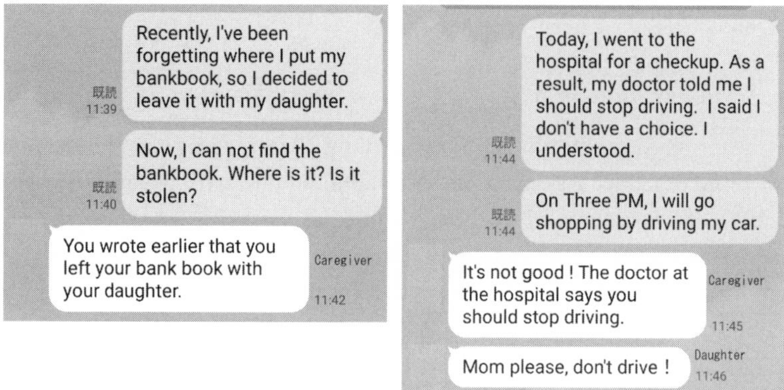

Figure 5-1 Support network system with LINE

linking with behind the ear-type transceivers. While travelling with family members or volunteers, a person with dementia is able to get quick support from the members just by talking to this system.

1.10 Telephones, frequent questions, and hearing impairment

Some family members suffer from frequent calls from persons with dementia. One of the ways to manage the frequent calls is to set up two phone numbers on their smartphone. One of the numbers is for the dedicated line between the person and the family member. They record answers to expected frequent questions there in advance. The persons can hear these recorded answers whenever they call, meanwhile the family members are not disturbed by their calls. Recently, you can have two phone numbers by installing some apps. Or several smartphones have this dual-phone number function. Ask your mobile carrier company for details.

The app "*U sound*" by Newbrick S.A. is a hearing aid app on a smartphone. With the app "*UD talk*" by Shamrock Records, speech is transcribed into text, and persons with a hearing impairment can read the text. Some apps have a function that enlarges the text on the screen and operates without the Internet. An app "*Mieru denwa* [visualized phone]" by NTT Docomo makes it possible to transcribe landline-caller's speech and show it on a smartphone in real time. You can exchange written messages remotely with people having hearing impairments if you use the app "*Tegaki denwa* [handwritten phone] *UD*" by Shamrock Records. You can also leave messages with this app so that family members, for instance, can respond to the other family's repetitive questions on the smartphones. If you use a tablet computer, you can show written messages in an enlarged font. This enlarged presentation is effective for people who refuse to wear hearing aids if the professional caregivers hang the tablet from the neck.

1.11 Hobbies and goggles for wearing smartphones

The "*Mezamashi doga* [wake-up video] *appli*" plays your favorite music and videos automatically at set times. Therefore, you can use the app as an intervention tool to perform music therapy and to have persons with dementia execute their daily routine by music (described in Chapter 6). If you install "*Karaoke JOYSOUND+*" by XING, you can sing while watching the lyrics. It also evaluates your singing with a score. The app "*Magic Piano*" made by Smule, plays classical/movie music and other kinds of music when the user taps rings falling from the top to the bottom of the screen. There are many instrument playing apps such as guitar, drums, xylophone, etc. Game playing is a desirable mental change for the elderly. "*Fusenwari* [balloon popping]" by CoCoPaPa Soft is an app for relieving stress by breaking balloons on the screen of your smartphone with your fingers. There are internet-communities where you can interact with others who have the same hobbies. "*DOKONOKO*" by Hobonichi is an app where many pictures of dogs and cats are posted every day, and you can interact with other pet lovers through comments. Goggles for wearing smartphones cost around 10 dollars. You can enjoy a more realistic game-playing environment by combining it with a headset. Various contents such as movies and tourist destinations in the world are being prepared. Some contents allow you to talk to digital players on the screen.

1.12 Other app programs

The app "*Alarm calendar Plus*" by Moyou enables your smartphone to tell you dates automatically by voice. You can use it as an alarm clock, too. Some persons with dementia lose their orientation for time and wait for several hours for a car to pick them up when they go, for instance, to the day-care center. With the app program "*Time keeper*" by Rossal04, your smartphone can inform you how many hours you have before you go out. Password management is becoming more difficult, even for healthy younger people. "*Password manager*" by Trend Micro can manage passwords and produce new passwords. Like children, some elderly people will use their smartphones for many hours. "*UBhind*" by RinaSoft allows a user to lock his/her smartphone at a predetermined time. Some apps can read and upload product names and prices on the Cloud when you take a picture of the receipts. These apps can also check the paid amount of your credit card.

The usability of the apps described so far depends on the individual's abilities and interests. It is important to find the programs best suited to their condition. Other apps can be found by searching websites with the keywords such as "recommended apps for the elderly" or "apps for surveillance and caring." Tokyo Information Technology Regional Support Center for Persons with Disabilities is releasing information about popular apps for persons with disabilities.

1.13 A smartphone case-holder with memo-pad

You cannot put pens, sticky-notes, or scratch paper in the commercially available case-holders for smartphones, yet they have pockets for cards. Several years ago, I modified a smartphone case-holder by attaching clear plastic pockets for sticky-notes and scratch paper. A tubular ring made of rubber was also fixed for carrying a pen (Figure 5-2). It might be better to hang this around your neck or to place it in your pocket, since your shoulders might become stiff from hanging things on them all day. With this "hybrid memo-pad," you can take notes easily, can pay by digital cards, and can access various information on the smartphone as well as answering and calling on the phone. Examples of the modified case-holder are shown on my website.

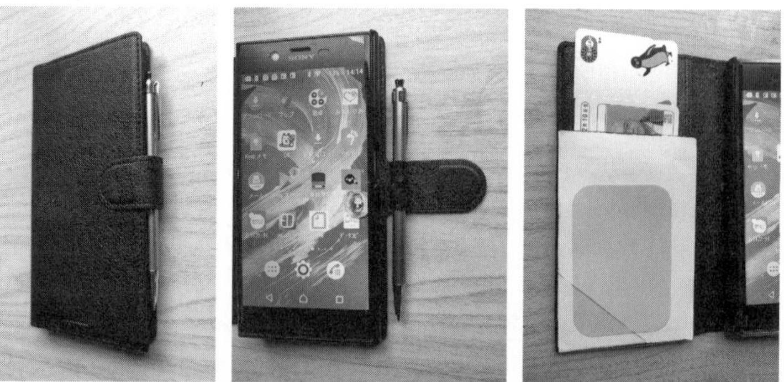

Figure 5-2 Memo-pad created by remodeling smartphone case-holder

1.14 Others

Recently, companies selling smartphones began to offer discount services to users with disabilities. Cost-saving smartphones are also becoming available today. Procedures to buy such smartphones on the Internet, however, are a little complicated. You may use services that will give you advice remotely on how to use your phone for 5 dollars per month. Private schools offer special classes for the elderly on how to use smartphones. The fee will be around 50 dollars monthly, and some schools offer private lessons at the customer's home. You may attend lessons for using a PC/smartphone at a nearby community center. You could organize a working group with your friends, inviting volunteers to teach smartphone operation. There is the Information Technology Regional Support Center for Persons with Disabilities in Tokyo and they provide advice and also hold training classes. Similar centers are available in all prefectures. Make contact with the local centers nearby and receive advice from them. My colleagues and I also hold the "Consultation Café for PC/smartphones" monthly at the regional community center (see Section 2.3 in Chapter 8).

1.15 Summary of support by using a smartphone

It is important to pick up a smartphone after its alarm sound goes off in the morning and to charge the phone at night (an alarm for this can be programmed on the smartphone). Even if you learned how to use your phone, you might forget it if you do not use it regularly. You should set alarms regularly for specified days and on those days practice using your smartphone with your friends and family. It is not always easy to learn how to use a smartphone even for the healthy elderly. However, once they have learned it, they will find it helpful to use, especially if they experience MCI or dementia later.

Figure 5-3 shows the card with notes used by an 85-year-old person with dementia who managed to learn how to use a cellphone with this card. Hopefully, applications (apps) will be developed which are dedicated to persons with MCI and dementia so that they can use smartphones with minimal effort. The government should fund the development of apps that help them maintain their independence. We should also consider recycling smartphones and starting a lending service for the elderly. The best apps would be installed on the loaned smartphone as well as the provision of training courses. These apps and services could reduce the cost of nursing

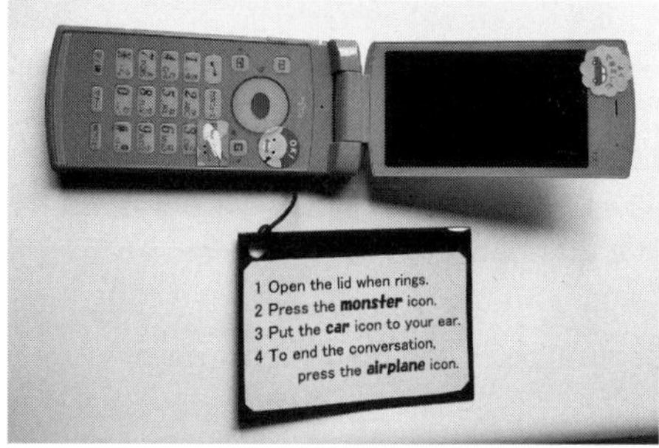

Figure 5-3 Tag with notes on how to use a cellphone

care insurance and delay admission to the elderly facility.

2. Clothing and others

In order to lead your daily life as desired, you should use several ATs described so far, such as memo-pads, the Sony IC Recorder (ICD-PX240; IC Rec), smartphones and so on. However, persons with MCI and dementia often forget to carry the ATs with them. Wearing special clothing that stores ATs inside pockets could solve these problems. Although there is no such clothing to purchase in the marketplace, instructions for sewing vests, aprons, and wheelchair bags with clear pockets for storing a memory book or wallet are available (Bourgeois, 2014). I conducted a project to develop assistive clothing with the laboratory of Utako Shimane at Wayo Women's University. The term "memory" was attached to all the names of assistive clothing produced in this project.

2.1 Memory vest

Persons with MCI and dementia often forget that they have a memo-pad with them. Or some of them find it troublesome to take a memo-pad out of their bags or pockets. They might forget also to take the smartphone, the IC Rec and other items with them. To address the need for persons with dementia to carry ATs with them and use them easily, we came up with the idea that they should wear a vest since a vest is available at a low price, easy to put on, and wearable throughout the year. It is also easy to add pockets or other modifications to the vest for the ATs.

The memory vests we created, which may be worn outside, are for the

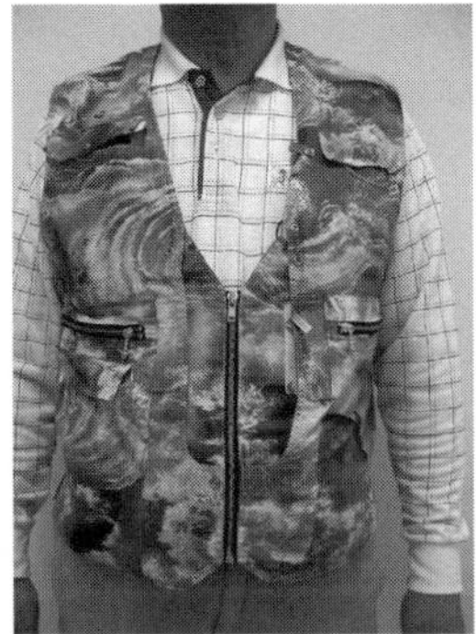

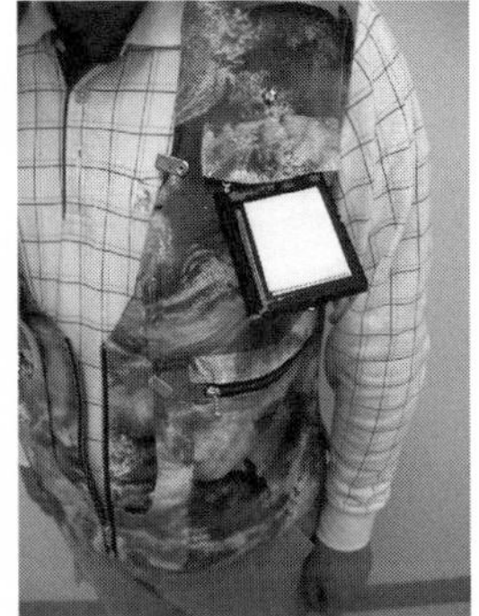

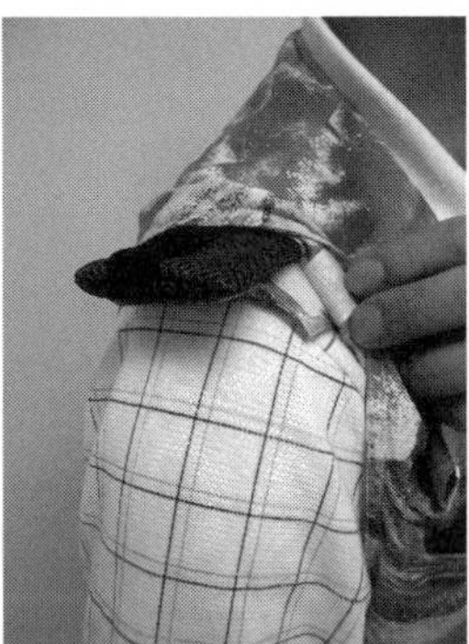

Figure 5-4 Memory vest

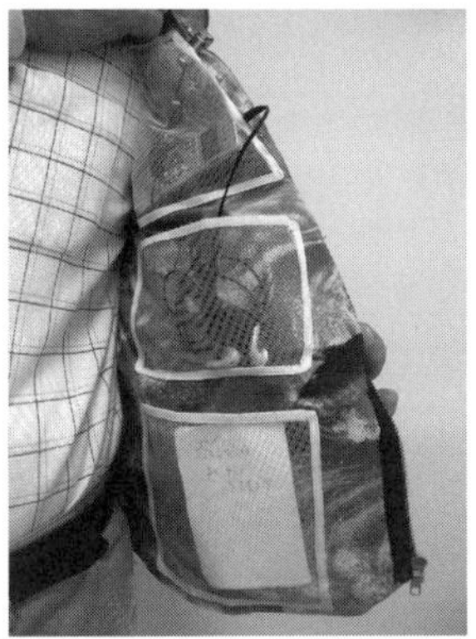

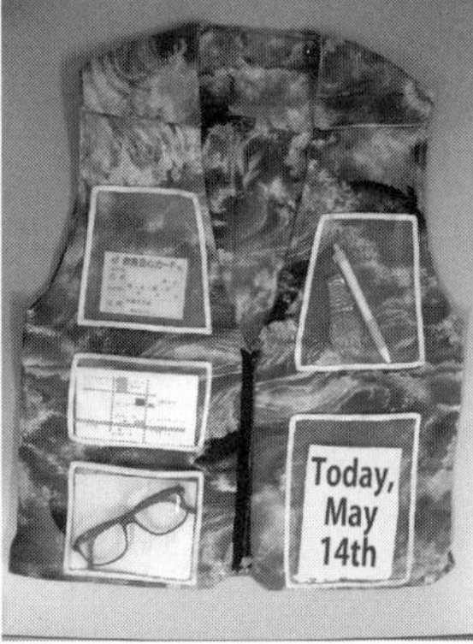

Figure 5-5 Reverse side of memory vest

healthy elderly, persons with MCI and with mild/moderate dementia. Wearing the vests, users can store and carry the ATs, IC Rec, as well as glasses, wallet, and keys. Some ATs can be operated without taking them out of pockets. As Figure 5-4 shows, you can use a compact-style message board (see Section 2.9 in Chapter 2) and a smartphone even without holding them. A shoulder pad of the vest can be changed into a tag with GPS when they start having trouble getting lost outside. On the reverse side of the vest, you can find several pockets made of mesh materials in various sizes. The merit of mesh pockets is that they are almost transparent and washable unlike vinyl pockets. In the mesh pockets, they may insert paper with messages on them such as, "It's ×× day, today" and "It's the day to go to the day-care center." They can see them when they open the front part of the vest (Figure

5-5). In other words, by putting on the vest they can wear "information."

Persons with moderate dementia forget where they have put memo-paper, then ask repeatedly where it is every several minutes. In such a case, family members may have persons wear the vest inside out if they agree to. Then they can see anytime what are in the pockets such as memo paper, devices, etc. (Figure 5-5). When they go out, or visitors come, they can put something on the vest, or reverse back the vest. Users can decide what they put in the vest pockets depending on their situation and necessity. This memory vest is also named "*Kanreki vest*" for observing users' 60th birthday, as people celebrate when turning 60 years old in Japan and it seems to be a suitable time to begin wearing it.

We have created three versions of memory vests: for winter, summer, and for year-round. The summer version is made of mesh material. The dress pattern of the year-round version is on my website (search with "Kiyoshi Yasuda homepage"). Please download and sew it, or take it to a dress-making shop. Nowadays, you can also search for sewing volunteers online. Although women's vests usually have few pockets, you can find vests for women with pockets in catalogs or online shops. If you want more pockets on your vest, you can sew mesh pockets on the reverse side of the vest. Many thanks to Miyoko Nagae, Kinuko Kagami, Mineko Aizawa, Tomoko Mineshima, and Mizuho Takahashi for sewing these vests.

2.2 Other clothing

Work shirts usually have large pockets on both fronts and so you can use them as "memory shirts." You may remove the flaps on the upper end of the pockets to make it easy to take the memo-pad/smartphone out and attach strings with clips to prevent dropping them. Users are recommended to put several clips on their pockets and to connect them to items such as a wallet or a smartphone by stretchable cords (see Section 2.3 in this chapter). Short sleeve work shirts should also be prepared for the summer.

People may find their neck getting stiff when they put many items in their vests. A pair of cargo pants that have pockets on both sides may be a good idea to alleviate stiffness caused by the weight of the vest. Short cargo pants are good for summer. A pair of pants called "*Suwaru* [sitting] *pants*" made by Value Innovation has pockets designed to let a user take items out of the pockets even in a sitting position. For very hot days, I created "memory trunks" for men with two smartphone pockets on both sides of the waist. Smartphone pockets are also available at dollar stores that can be attached to the top edge of trunks with two clips.

A man with MCI in his 90s suggested that the elderly should wear black trunks, since black-colored clothes do not show stains clearly even when an accident happens. Currently, many trunks and shorts that absorb urine leakage are on the market. These products let you continue your outing. It is the family member's burden to dress the elderly with cognitive and physical impairment due to the rigidity and involuntary movements of the limbs. "*Nobinobi* [stretchy] *one touch hadagi* [underwear]" is extremely stretchy and easy to put on (Figure 5-6). "*Ryowaki* [both side] *zenkai* [fully open] *sweat pants*" by Kaunet allow both sides of the pants to fully open (Figure 5-7). This helps family members change diapers while a person is standing or assist a person to put on the pants while he/she is sitting.

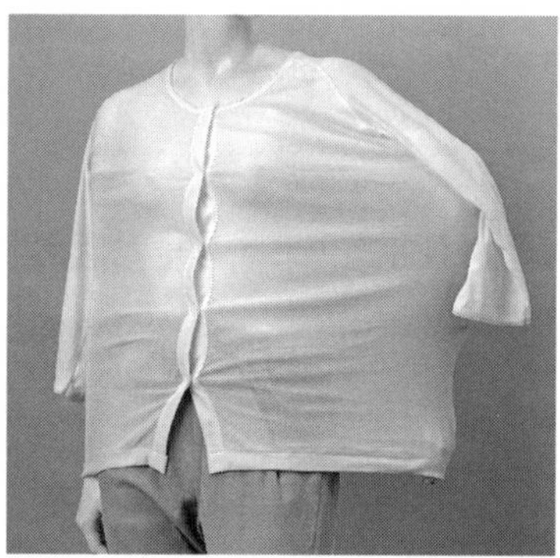

Figure 5-6 *Nobinobi* [stretchy] *one touch hadagi* [underwear]
Source: Francebed, https://medical.francebed.co.jp/kaigoyouhinonline/item/92141700.html.

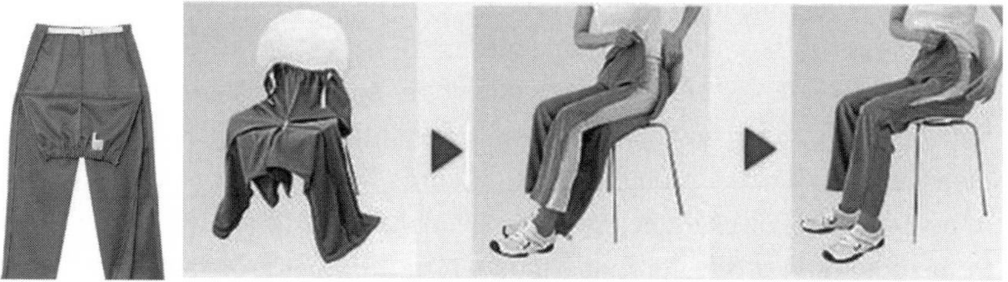

Figure 5-7 *Ryowaki* [both side] *zenkai* [fully open] *sweat pants*
Source: Kaunet, https://www.kaunet.com/rakuraku/variation/00037239/.

Related Topics —Video recording of activities during the day—

If you could video-tape all the activities during the day, it would become useful when searching for your belongings or retrieving what you talked about. This led us to an important system of ATs for persons with MCI and dementia. As described in Yasuda, Nakamura, Kuwahara et al. (2011), the IC Recorder (IC Rec) automatically emitted the following instructions every morning for a man with MCI. At first the recorded message told him to wear the memory vest, then attach to it one of the three small cameras prepared in advance. The cameras were for wide-angle video-taping and recorded the scene in front of him, i.e., the faces and voices of the people. Additionally, he was asked to wear the IC Rec and to record on it by speaking about what he was doing. Due to the shortage of the camera's battery, the message from the IC Rec also asked him to exchange the camera three times a day and to charge it each time. One day, wearing these ATs he went shopping with a notice on the front pocket "Now, recording for daily-life support." He succeeded in recording 11 hours of video and voices during the day. Recorded voices on the IC Rec were transcribed into texts. Time stamps for each voice input were automatically attached like, "[9:35] I am going to the market to buy milk." The time stamp was used as a clue to search for a specific scene on the video later on. Problems encountered with this system were the short battery-life and recording other peoples' faces on the video. If we could solve these problems, for example, by means of auto video-recording only when needed to save the batteries and of mosaicking the faces automatically, this system would become more practical. Fortunately, recent smartphones have a wide-angle video-camera. The smartglasses, which will be described later, can be another alternative method for this system.

2.3 Memory handbag

Persons with dementia often leave their bags behind when out in the community. For information about the alarm device to use on a handbag, see Section 1.4 in Chapter 4. In the case that the device is not available, hanging the bag on the shoulder diagonally may help them to not remove the bag from their body and misplace their bags so often. The elderly tend to put too many items in their bags, and they often have difficulty finding their necessary items promptly. Elastic cords in different colors are useful in many ways. For example, they can tie a blue cord to the wallet, tie a clip to the other end of the cord, and then put the clip onto the bag. When they want to take the wallet out from the bag, for example, they pull the blue cord (Figure 5-8).

A handbag called "*Ramukawa takinou tesage* [multi-purpose lamb-

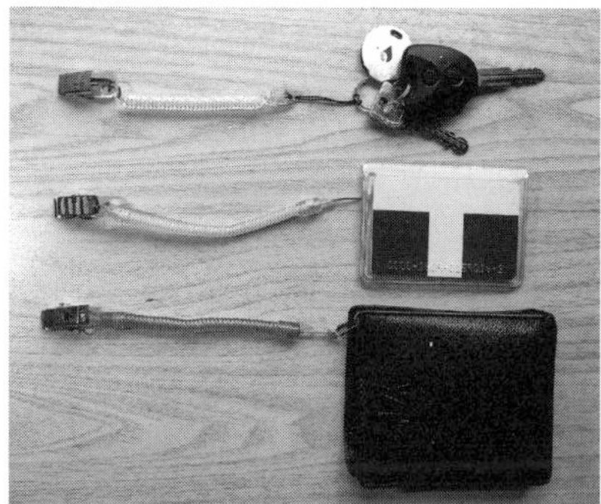

Figure 5-8 Cords with clips for keeping items safe and handy

leather] *bag*" by Yuri Kojima and a book-style clear file, "*Inner document file*" by Lihit Lab, to be put into handbags are on the market, and using the above bag and the file together is useful for organizing items inside bags and is helpful for finding items in bags; we may call it a "Memory handbag." If you have many bags, you might forget in which bag you put a certain item. Thus, it is advisable to choose a bag you like the best and only use that bag. Or, select a small (inner) bag to put small items in, and then put it into a bigger (outer) bag. This system is called "Bag-in-bag." You can choose a favorite outer bag when you go out without changing the inner bag.

2.4 Memory waist bag and memory pouch

Figure 5-9 shows "memory bag" to which a memo-pad and the IC Recorder are attached by magnets to the commercially available waist bag. This bag

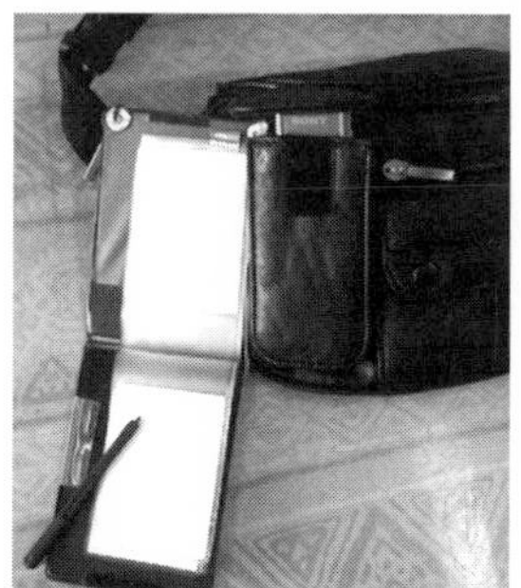

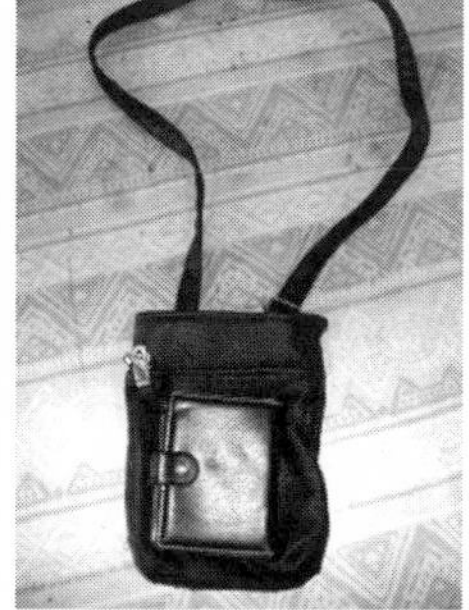

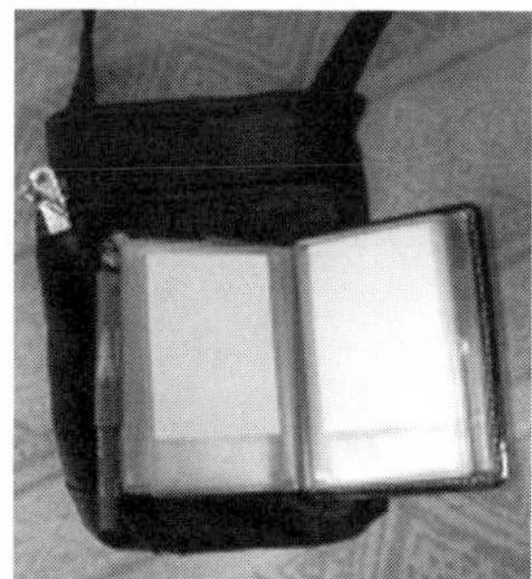

Figure 5-9 Memory waist bag and memory pouch

allows you to take notes easily and to record your thoughts on the IC Rec while walking. A type of bag called a "security pouch" is also useful. The bag is usually used as a travel bag in which you put a passport and travel items, and you can hang it from your neck. To make it a "memory pouch," a memo-pad has been attached to the bag by magnets or Velcro tape.

2.5 Memory hanging pockets

If you place your belongings (such as memo-pads, letters, documents, medicines, medical cards, your glasses, and so forth) everywhere you like, you will spend a lot of time looking for them every day. Figure 5-10 is "memory hanging pockets" into which you can put the belongings you use regularly and hang it on the wall. The top part of the hanging pockets is for medicines, memo-pads, and pens-and-pencils. The digital clock is for checking dates. If you replace the clock with a tablet computer, you can use it as a videophone device, and your family members can communicate with you and check remotely whether you have taken your medicines. In this case, a bottle of water should be hung so that you can take medicine in front of the camera.

You may use a memo-board on which magnet sheets are attached with messages such as, "It's the day to go to the day-care center." You can keep

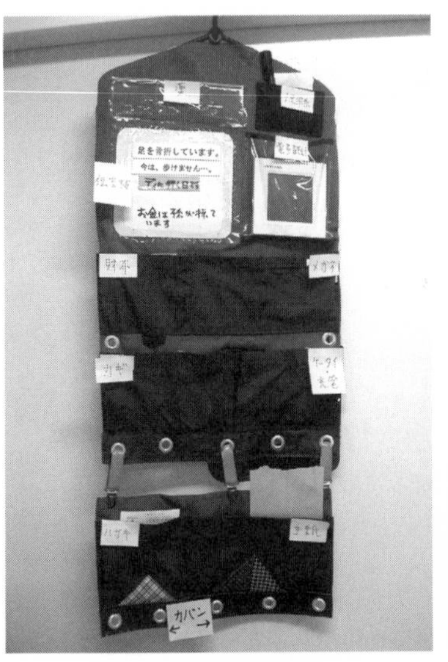

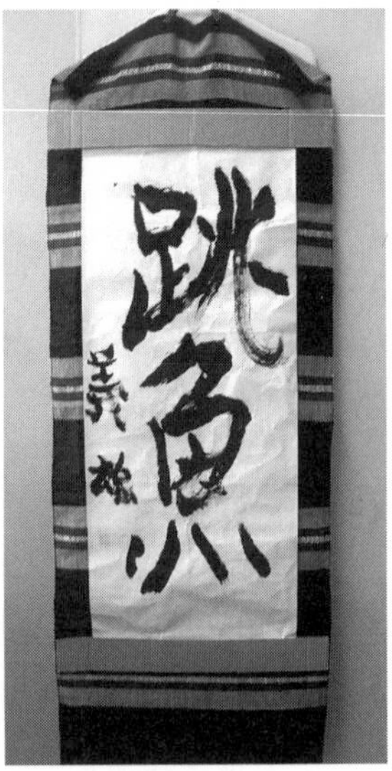

Figure 5-10 Memory hanging pockets

your smartphone and charge it inside the pocket if an electronic cord extends into the pocket from the wall outlet behind the hanging pockets. The eyelets at the bottom are used to hang bags with S-hooks. In order to draw the user's attention to the hanging pockets, you can put photos (e.g., of your favorite person) on it. You can use a clock or an IC Rec to output messages or alarms regularly to draw attention to the information on the magnet board, such as "Here is today's plan."

If you attach a name card to each pocket, it will help you check at a glance what belongings are missing from the pockets. The hanging pockets are ideal to use together with a medicine calendar. The hanging pockets should be transparent. Various types of the hanging pockets or wall pockets are sold at dollar stores or on the website. You may freely combine these pockets. It will be convenient to hang them at the entrance of your house or your room. When you go out and you come back, you put your belongings in the pockets to prevent your belongings from being scattered. If you do not want to show the hanging pockets to visitors, cover it with a sheet. Or turn it and show its back, which could be decorated with an embroidery or calligraphy (Figure 5-10). If you have difficulty in reaching items overhead, side storage cabinets are usable as a "memory box" which can be set under or beside a table.

2.6 Memory table

Due to age-related cognitive decline/impairment and the increase of personal belongings over time, some elderly people have difficulty in organizing belongings, even the things on their tables. If drawers are fixed on the table, it may help the elderly know the whereabouts of their belongings. Drawer sets (Figure 5-11) are available at dollar stores (e.g., "Seria A5 drawer's Box," by SPOON HOME). These drawers are fixed on the table and covered by a plate. In this way, drawers can be pulled out under the cover plate. If you use several boards to make the cover plate, items such as stationery and letters in the drawers can be quickly taken out by folding the cover plates (Figure 5-12). If you make the cover plate transparent or translucent, all items can be seen and checked at any time. To accommodate the increased height of the table, the height of the chair should be raised accordingly. It will become more convenient if you use the side drawers introduced in Section 6 of Chapter 2 together with this table. When visitors come, you may cover the table with a tablecloth. In the future, I would expect furniture makers to create furniture that is elderly-friendly.

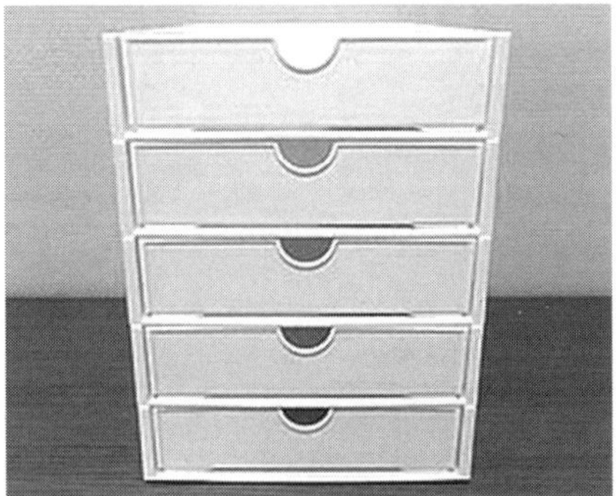

Figure 5-11 Drawer sets

Source: Pinterest, https://www.pinterest.jp/pin/808044358121884215/.

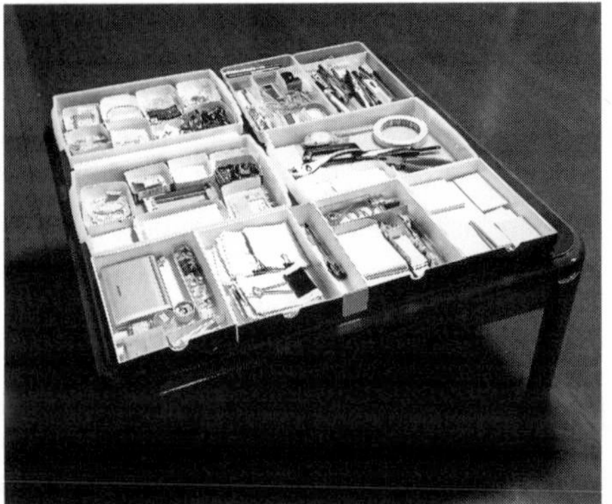

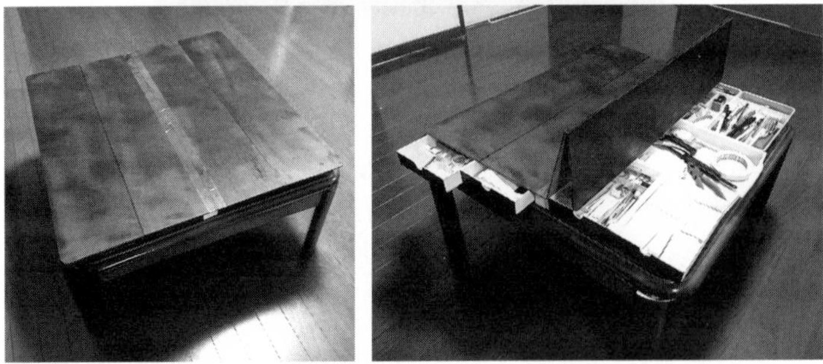

Figure 5-12 Drawers on a table and covered by a plate

CHAPTER SIX

Psychological and communication support using therapeutic applications of AT

In these days, reminiscence therapy, music therapy, and other non-pharmacological interventions are employed for the residents and users of elder facilities. These interventions may relieve their challenging problems and activate their communicative motivation. In this chapter, several kinds of interventions, particularly using Middle-Tech ATs are outlined. The evidence levels for these interventions are still low (Japanese Society of Neurology, 2017). The levels, however, are expected to rise if professionals in this field accumulate their experiences and research using these interventions, while selecting interventions that are the best suited for each person with MCI/ dementia.

1. Reminiscence therapy

Reminiscence therapy is one of the approaches suggested in order to increase feelings of positive self-esteem and psychosocial well-being, and to decrease behavioral disturbances (Yasuda, Kuwahara, Abe et al., 2009). Despite degeneration of short-term memory function, persons with dementia often retain a facility for long-term memory. Reminiscence therapy is a means of stimulating long-term memory to prompt communication in persons with dementia (Gowans, Campbell, Alm et al., 2004).

1.1 Materials for reminiscence therapy

When the stage of dementia becomes more severe, persons may not be able to understand the meaning of discourse, sentences, or even words. Consequently, some persons with severe dementia may feel anxious and stressed all the time. If they are given something to enjoy and concentrate on for a certain period of time, their challenging problems may be reduced. Reminiscence therapy is an intervention which is often applied to persons with mild to severe dementia. Recently, various photos for reminiscence therapy are available on the market. For example, "*Shashinde miru nihon seikatsu zuhiki* [photos of Japanese daily life]" by Koubunsha, "*Puromaido kaiso* [reminiscence pictures of the celebrity]" by Trendmaster, and "*Shouka karuta*" (a collection of pictures for playing games while listening to songs by CD) by Hatachi are available for purchase.

Today, you can also search for free photos suitable for reminiscence therapy on the Internet. The "NHK (Japan Broadcasting Cooperation) Archives" offers a website "Reminiscence Library" for free. On this website, you can watch various old movies and TV programs from the 1940-60's, pictures of old tools, customs, songs, living styles, local news, school activities, and more. Some contents are accompanied with simple questions which let viewers talk about their memories, and some are edited for VR goggles.

Meanwhile, if you search by a keyword, for example "rugby player" for the rugby fans on the Internet and then click on "images," you can find many related photos. You can talk with the fans while watching these photos for a while. When persons with dementia are restless at the waiting room in a hospital, family members can show them their favorite photos on the Internet. Otake (2012) proposed a group reminiscence therapy in which each member brings her/his photos to the gathering and the members show their photos in turn and talk about the photos.

The Showa Era Life-Style Museum in Kitanagoya City exhibits a huge number of daily goods, devices, posters, and other tools used in the *Showa* period (i.e., 1926–1989). In persons' homes, family members may set up a reminiscence corner with old types of goods, posters, and furniture that they might feel comforting. Yamazaki (2008–2009) set up a reminiscence corner at home where old photo albums could be easily looked at when his mother with dementia stopped by (Figure 6-1). Yamazaki (2015) also proposed a virtual Buddhist altar as an application program for reminiscence therapy on tablet computers. On the monitor, users can see *ihai* (memorial tablets) with incense and the photo of the deceased. They may participate remotely in a funeral ceremony. In the near future persons with dementia may be able to talk with avatars of the deceased on the monitor and to get advice about their daily lives from them. The effects of these types of reminiscence

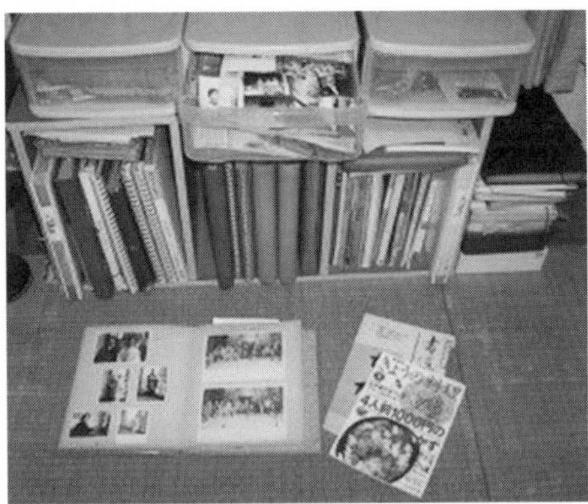

Figure 6-1 Reminiscence therapy corner

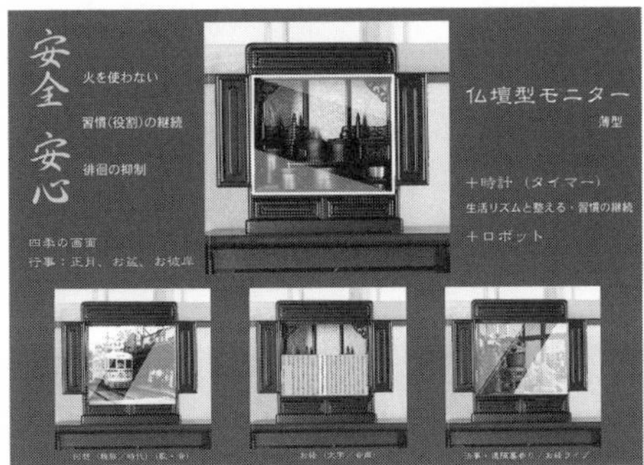

Figure 6-2 Buddhist altar on monitor

therapies will need to be evaluated as they are developed. (Figure 6-2).

Recently, projectors are small enough to fit in the palm, and users can project photos /videos through it on the wall from smartphones or PCs; this may let users feel as if they are watching movies in a movie theater. There are also projectors with a ceiling light function from which visual images can be projected onto the wall. This system may be effective for persons who become restless at night, or persons with Lewy body dementias who see hallucinations on the wall.

1.2 Videos for reminiscence therapy

Around 1997, a reminiscence video series for persons with dementia were sold in the U.S.A. (Lund, Hill, Caserta et al., 1995). In the videos performers showed photos and old items, and talked slowly about topics that were likely to be favored by them. Referring to these videos, Yasuda (2008a) produced "*Katarikake* [talking] *video*" DVDs. On the DVDs you can listen to old songs and reminiscence about the songs. Some professionals at care-facilities commented on the DVDs, saying that the songs were easy for elderly listeners to hear because a male singer sings slowly in a low pitch. In order to watch these videos for an extended period of time, however, sustained attention and concentration are required. These videos have been shown to be empirically effective for persons with mild and moderate dementia (Lund et al., 1995).

A DVD called "*Pasokon kaisoho* [reminiscence therapy on PC]" by N-Progress shows old tools and scenes with written explanations and questions on the monitor. Another DVD "*Natsukashino tamatebako* [old treasure boxes]" by Silver Channel shows a collection of video images of old tools, traditional and seasonal customs, and more. Usually, reminiscence therapy is conducted at facilities under the guidance of professionals. But persons with dementia can enjoy these DVDs to reminisce and sing even at home alone.

1.3 Personalized reminiscence photo videos

Despite its effectiveness, regular reminiscence intervention is often difficult to perform, especially at home, due to a shortage of human resources. Therefore, home-oriented reminiscence interventions should be provided (Yasuda, Kuwabara, Kuwahara et al., 2009). As the stages of dementia progress, persons with severe dementia may lose interest in the videos mentioned in the previous section, due to fading general/social knowledge of traditional tools, events and so on. On the other hand, their personal memories may be preserved still. For such persons, therefore, we developed the

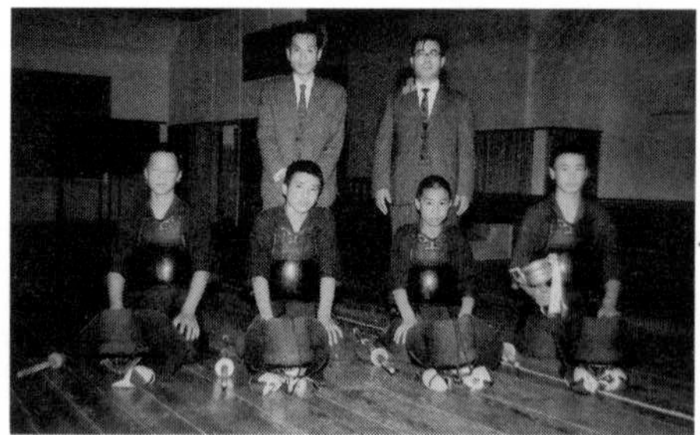

Figure 6-3 Personalized reminiscence photo video

personalized reminiscence photo video called "*Omoide shashin* [reminiscent photo] *video*" (Figure 6-3) (Yasuda et al., 2009). Each video contains 50 to 100 photos of the individual, which are recorded on CDs or DVDs. Each photo was shown about 15 seconds and accompanied with brief narration. The completed video for each individual lasts approximately 30 to 40 minutes. Two volunteer companions participated in the project; one of them took videos and edited them. To make the interaction more engaging, a pan/zoom effect was added to the video.

Another companion recorded narration with a slow and gentle voice on each photo. In order to not induce stress from difficulty of recalling memories, the volunteer narrator was asked to avoid detailed questions, such as, "Where was this photograph taken?", and "Who is sitting next to you?" Because, the persons with dementia often lack correct autobiographical memories. Instead, the narrator frequently praised them in the photographs, saying for example, "You look beautiful", and "Your dress is very nice", or the narrator made confirmative descriptive statements, such as, "They are eating a delicious meal." Since old music and children's songs are effective for attracting persons (Yasuda et al., 2006a), such music is played in the background to increase their enjoyment.

In our experiment (Yasuda et al., 2009), 12 participants were classified into three groups: mild, moderate, and severe dementia. They were asked to watch their own reminiscent photo video twice and each of the TV shows (news and variety show) once in an ABCA design. The total length was 40 minutes. Each of the participants watched the four shows in a room by him or herself. Their behaviors were recorded on videotape. Their responses were evaluated independently by three speech pathologists. Responses were measured in terms of concentration (e.g., nodding, laughing, etc.) and distraction scores (sleeping, looking away, etc.).

The results revealed that the photo videos are effective in helping participants with dementia focus their concentration. Moreover, the photo video may be effective for participants, especially with moderate and severe dementia, whereas the TV news and the TV variety show seemed to be less effective for maintaining concentration for them (Figure 6-4).

The mild group showed poor concentration for the second photo video presentation (2A in Figure 6-4). Our interpretation is that they remembered the photos in the first presentation and were bored by seeing the same photos 30 minutes later. In contrast, the moderate and severe group showed concentration scores for the second photo video that were much higher than

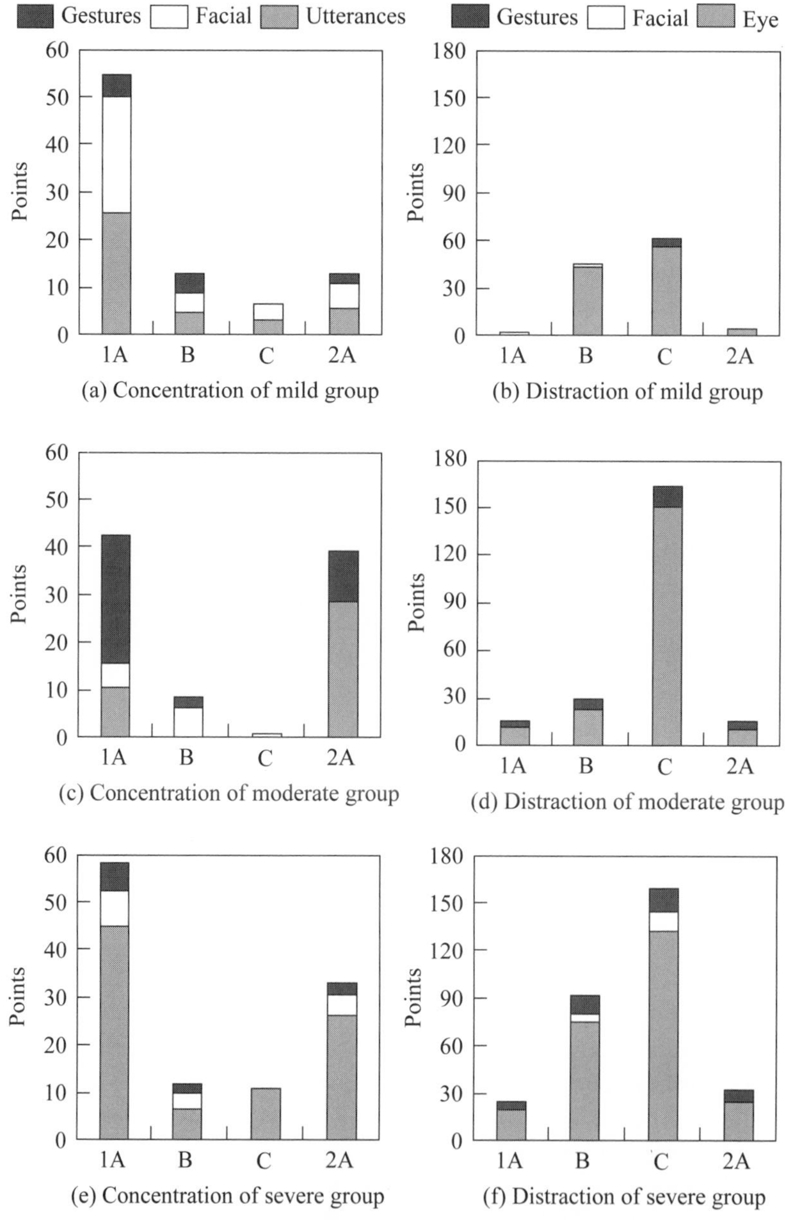

Figure 6-4 Experiment using personalized reminiscence photo videos

Note: 1A = 1st photo video, B = TV variety show, C = TV news show, 2A = 2nd photo video.

those shown by the mild group.

The severe group's distraction scores (f) increased considerably for the TV variety show, compared to those of the mild (b) and moderate group participants (d). Participants in the severe group already have difficulty enjoying even the TV variety show (Lund et al., 1995). The photo video appears to be an appropriate method to attract their attention. Some participants gave extensive oral responses to the video. Thus, the video may work as a prompter of verbal communication for some participants.

The son of a woman with severe dementia introduced the following episode to us, "My mother seems to have returned to her former self after watching her reminiscence photo video." She watched her video with joy and tears every day for three years. She was unable to remember the fact that she saw it the day before, therefore, she did not get tired of watching the same video for three years.

Persons with dementia sometimes display the delusion of jealousy and abuse their family members. This is probably because they recall only bad episodes about their family members. The person mentioned above had also been verbally abusing her husband. But while watching her reminiscence photo video and after that, such abuse always disappeared. Further, she talked intimately to her husband after she watched the video. This happened probably because the video helped her remember the times when she lived in harmony with her husband. A man exhibited a big smile after he watched his reminiscence photo video though he was always angry at the people around him. The video is a type of complementary intervention in having viewers recall pleasant memories especially for those who tend to recall unpleasant memories of the past. Today, you can watch photos together remotely with your family if you use the "share screen" function of videophones.

There are companies on the Internet that can digitize photos onto DVDs, for which there is an editing cost. To make a personalized reminiscence photo video all at once without editing cost and procedures, you take videos of the photos with a handy video camera or a smartphone and simultaneously record narration on the episode for each photo while playing old songs as background music.

Such recorded videos can be transferred onto SD cards or DVDs to play on DVD players, or tablets. Many digital photo frames show videos by just turning the switch on. It is also advisable to show the video at times when persons with dementia are likely to refuse going to the hospital or day-care

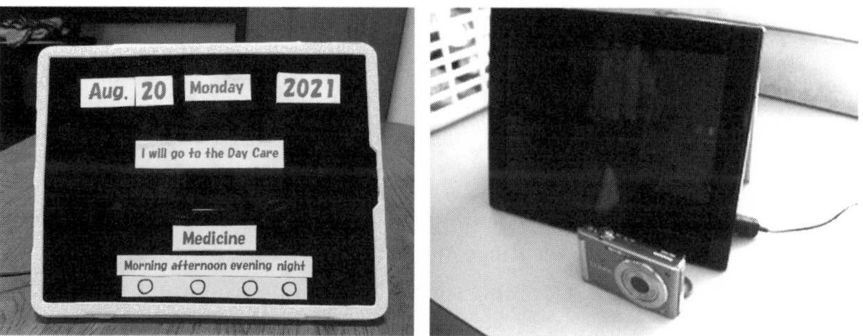

Figure 6-5 Digital photo frame

center. A digital photo frame "*KD8JV-S*" by Keian automatically starts showing videos at a set time. If the personalized reminiscence photo video is played automatically, it could be effective for preventing responsive behaviors at a fixed time, such as every evening when they feel restless and feel like going back to their "old" home (also known as "sundown syndrome"). As many family members tend to forget to play the videos when necessary, the automatic playing feature is very helpful in order to execute **the strategy of presenting information in advance**. The picture at the left of Figure 6-5 is a message board for written memos that covers the photo frame. When videos are shown, the message board raises up (Figure 6-5).

Some digital photo frames allow for recorded verbal messages. For example, "*Message photo album*" by Intel Giken enables you to record 10 second messages for each of 72 photos. A pen called "*Act voice pen*" by Escor can play a recorded message if you put the pen close to an electric sticker stuck to each photo. If you record on the pen questions and comments such as, "They are playing a watermelon splitting game,"it becomes a tool for

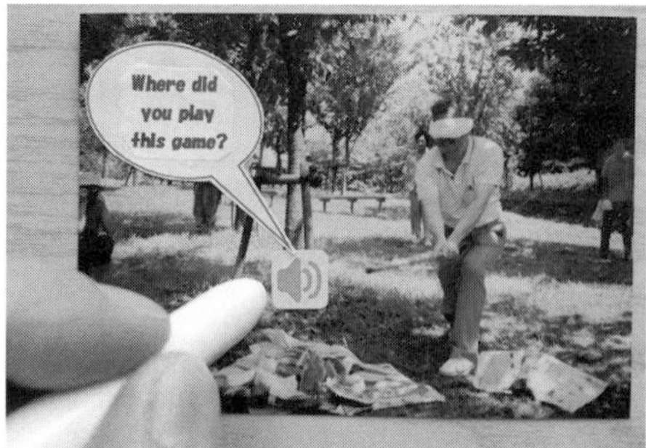

Figure 6-6 Reminiscence therapy using "*Act voice pen*"

reminiscence therapy. You can also record the names of friends on each photo so that it can be used as a training device to recall their names. A micro-SD card can be inserted into the pen to record messages for five hours in total (Figure 6-6).

Bourgeois (2014) introduced electronic memory books which can have a caption or a recorded message to describe each picture. The "talking" memory book is particularly useful for persons with dementia for whom the voices of family members would be comforting. There are also applications available for use with the iPad to create a talking memory book that speaks aloud the sentences typed into each page. The pictures for the memory book are easily uploaded from users' electronic library files.

2. Music therapy

Music can calm, excite, persuade or inspire us, and lift our spirits especially when we are cognitively impaired (Foster, 2009). Musical abilities of individuals with dementia remain intact for an extended period of time, despite their cognitive deterioration (Ingram, 2012). Music therapy has no standard forms or contents. In institutions, participants often spend about one hour singing songs, playing musical instruments, doing body exercises with music (Oshima, Itou, Nishimoto et al., 2013).

2.1 Tempting persons with dementia to a day-care center by music

Persons with moderate and severe dementia often show low motivation for doing daily routines when they are instructed to do by family members. Sometimes, it is even harder to lead them into doing routines by recorded messages of the Sony IC Recorder (ICD-PX240; IC Rec). In order to raise their motivation, we conducted the following experiment in which music was played before the instructions were emitted (Yasuda, Beckman, Yoneda et al., 2006a). A person with Alzheimer's disease had often refused to go to the day-care center. Therefore, several songs were played for him before the center's car arrived to pick him up. The songs were old, cheerful, and rhythmical songs with the lyrics praising the mountains, the sea, and going out. The songs had been recorded onto the IC Rec and then were played automatically approximately 15 minutes before the car was scheduled to arrive. Together with the songs, the recorded instructions by the first author were played at the beginning and in the intervals of three songs (Yasuda et al., 2006a). The essence of the instructions was to ask him to prepare for

Table 6-1 Examples of music and verbal instructions by IC Rec

[At 8:25 on the day to go to the day-care center] Mr. ××, good morning! I am ×× of ×× hospital. Did you sleep well last night? How is the weather, today? Now, I will play an old song for you. (Title of song)
[Output the song. He hears the following messages before and after each song.] Isn't this a nice old song? (Then, some questions related to the song.) The next song is: (Title of song).
[While playing another song] Shall we go for a walk? You will feel better if you go out. [Repeat the songs. While playing the songs, he can get ready and a center's car will arrive to pick him up.]

going to the day-care center (see Table 6-1).

On the third day of the intervention, his wife came to the hospital to see us. We were worried that something had gone wrong, but she said to us with a big smile, "Success! I had never thought that such a childish trick would work, but it did. I wanted to report about it quickly." Figure 6-7 shows the stress levels felt by his wife before and after the intervention. The levels were based on her own self-assessment of the stress she felt during the process of sending her husband to the day-care center. She had almost no stress after the intervention began (level 1 means no stress).

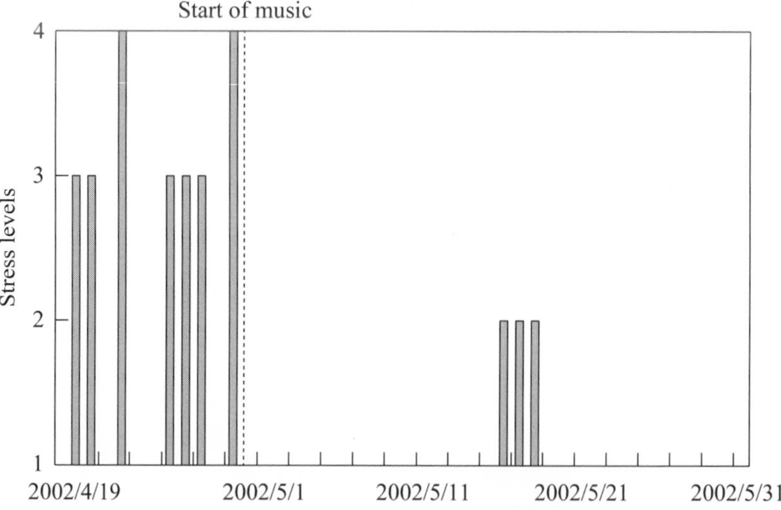

Figure 6-7 Levels of stress felt by wife

Note: 1 = no stress, 4 = high stress.

There are many persons with dementia who refuse to go to day-care centers, and this causes much stress for their family members. We tried this intervention with other persons and other routines, such as dressing, eating, and going to hospitals. The intervention worked well for 70–80 % of them although the period during which the intervention was effective was different for each person. An alternative idea is to record invitation messages, such as, "Please come to have a lunch with us. Your friend is waiting for you," onto the IC Rec. Family members may ask the staff members or participants who are friendly with him/her at the centers to record messages, and, if possible, to record the messages with music.

2.2 Morning music may lead to a calm day

Several weeks had passed after the person in the previous section began listening to music before going to the center. A member of staff told his wife that, "He has been calm at the center recently." We checked the communication notebooks about his behaviors. As Table 6-2 shows, six incidents of negative behaviors, such as, "Speaking harsh words," "Walking around" and others were reported in the 45 days before the person began listening to music in the morning, but only one negative behavior, "showing a grim face" was reported in the 45 days after the music intervention. There was no change in his circumstances including medications during this period. It is possible that listening to the music in the morning made his emotions stable and that the effect continued during the stay at the center and until evening, although he forgot that he listened to the music. Similar results have been reported in the Japanese Music Therapy Academy. These reports suggest that the effects of music are likely to last for long periods of time (Yasuda et al., 2006a).

Table 6-2 The person's problematic speech and behaviors in the day-care center (reported on the communication notebook)

45 days before listening to the music in the morning (March 18th–May 2nd)
Speaking harsh words to others temporarily
Walking around in the center
Talking in a displeased manner and showing nervous and stiff looks
Restless all day
Refusing to have his temperature taken, etc.
Keeping on moving in the center
45 days after listening to the music in the morning (May 3rd–June 17th)
Showing a grim face

2.3 Reducing anger by music

There was a person with cerebrovascular dementia who often got angry at his wife about something trivial. He even hit her with his walking stick sometimes. His doctor prescribed sedative pills, but he did not stop verbally abusing his wife. Meanwhile, he was often found eagerly listening to songs for school children in the Memory Clinic. Therefore, we asked an amateur music composer to select songs that would make him feel at ease. He compiled songs into four sets; (each set has three/four songs). We outputted automatically one of the four sets in turn from the IC Rec 10 times a day every day (Yasuda et al., 2006a). The IC Rec also output the greetings from the first author at the beginning and the end of each set. The greeting at the end was, "Please have a nice, relaxed day today." As a result, he seldom got angry, although previously he had become enraged every second or third day (Figure 6-8).

One day, while he was angry, the songs happened to start playing. Immediately, he bent his ear to the songs and then calmed down. When the songs stopped, he seemed to look forward to the next songs coming out. We gave him, therefore, a cassette tape of songs, so that he could listen to them anytime. His wife commented later saying, "Songs were more effective than medicine (Yasuda et al., 2006a)."

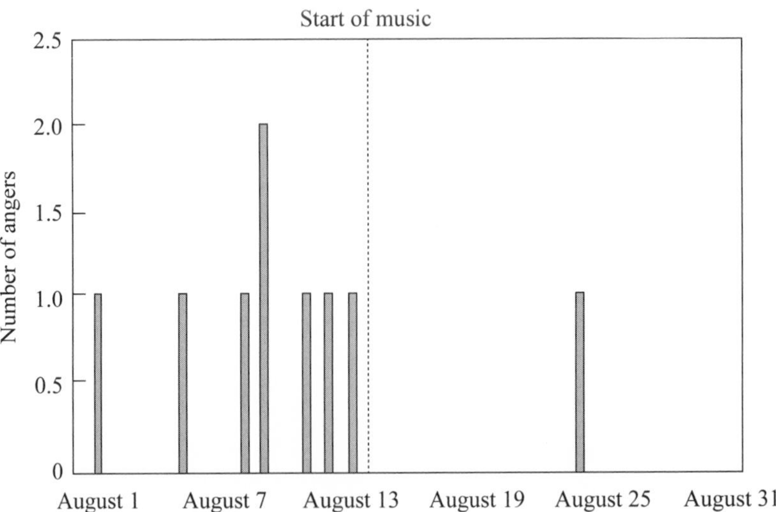

Figure 6-8 Number of angers reported by wife

2.4 Tempting persons with dementia to study, walk, and wake up by music

We advised a person who had aphasia after a cerebral stroke to practice writing *kanji* words at home, but she seldom did it. So, we outputted a verbal instruction, "Let's do the homework," from the IC Rec every day at regular times, but it did not work for her. Then, before the instruction in the IC Rec, we recorded two songs in order to inspire her to sing with them. As a result, the person, who had previously done the homework only two or three days a month, did the homework 25 days in a month after we implemented singing songs.

A person with Parkinson's disease seldom went for a walk because it took time to start the initial movement due to stiffness caused by the disease. We set the IC Rec to play songs for 15 minutes before his wife prompted him to go for a walk every day. At first, his starting movements were still slow and clumsy. Gradually, he started getting ready for walks by moving his body according to the songs. Persons with Lewy body dementia have syndromes similar to Parkinson's disease, so their movements may begin to slow down. The same intervention was applied to a person with Lewy body dementia and the frequency of her walks increased too.

The number of persons with dementia who live alone is increasing. Some of them complain more about being less motivated in the morning than about daily forgetfulness. For instance, some persons with dementia find it troublesome to change their clothes. In order to deal with such problems, I recorded my greetings and songs on the IC Rec, and replaced the alarm clocks with the IC Rec. In this way, the users were woken up by the voice saying, "Good morning," then heard songs, and finally listened to the message, "Let's get up and change your clothes!" Five or six persons who tried this intervention reported that they were motivated and got up smoothly. In the case of a woman who became less motivated in starting daily house chores after she had a subarachnoid hemorrhage, several songs were played to her before she was to do each household task.

Some persons with dementia develop sleep pattern irregularity caused by staying up late and in turn, having trouble getting up in the morning, or taking excessive daytime naps. It might be an idea worth trying to play a lullaby to encourage such persons to go to sleep.

2.5 Cases of songs being ineffective

Interventions by songs, however, are not always effective. There was a person with dementia who became very sensitive to the noise around him. For example, the sound of cars running by, or the voices of children playing outside were annoying to him. He became extremely restless when the wind was strong during typhoons. Thus, the music intervention was not applied for him. For another person, we outputted songs automatically from the IC Rec: the songs that he used to like before he had dementia. He showed, unexpectedly, a displeased look when he heard the songs, and so, we stopped trying this intervention. We also tried to have a person with visual hallucinations listen to a chorus of school songs at his home. However, he became confused with hearing the songs, believing that a choral group had come to his home to sing. We stopped an attempt of this intervention for him too. It is necessary to observe persons carefully before and after we introduce the music intervention.

2.6 Increasing appetite through music and dolls

A woman who suffered from severe Alzheimer's disease and cerebrovascular dementia lost her appetite and she ate on average only 10 to 20 % of the amount of food necessarily served to her. Meanwhile, when she visited the Memory Clinic, she showed an affection for dolls, and listened to children's songs for more than half an hour. Based on this observation, we speculated that outputting music and voice messages from a doll could increase her appetite (Yasuda et al., 2006a). On the IC Rec, we recorded a total of about 40 minutes of messages and songs. The lyrics of the songs were changed to stimulate her appetite such as, "Today, we are having a feast. It is delicious," "We are having newly harvested rice," and "You used to be scolded if you left some food on your plate." The songs were played and sung by a piano teacher. The messages were inserted between songs. The IC Rec was hidden in the back of the doll. The doll was placed on the dining table and the songs and messages were outputted automatically from the doll at dinner time every night.

She responded to almost all the messages, crying for joy and clapping along with the songs while she was eating dinner. Consequently, she began eating on average up to 50 % of the food she was served two weeks after the intervention was introduced (Yasuda et al., 2006a). The appetite of healthy people also likely increased if they eat while talking with friends

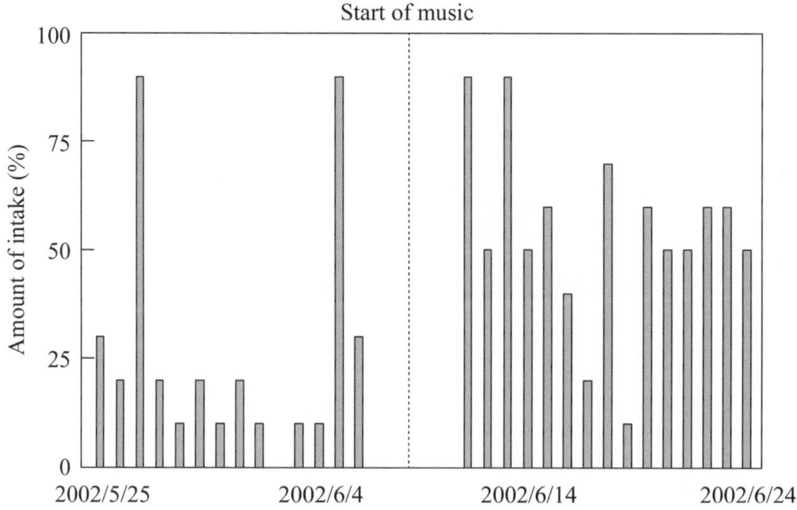

Figure 6-9 Amount of food intake

and listening to music. Similar effects seemed to be achieved by using a doll and the IC Rec in the above intervention (Figure 6-9).

Related Topics —**Development of a suction toothbrush and an oral light**—
When the stage of dementia has progressed to severe, persons often become unable to clean their teeth. Furthermore, they often refuse to open their mouth for cleaning. At this stage, aspiration pneumonia could occur. Although it is important to clean the oral cavity of persons, it can be difficult as they sometimes bite their family members' or professional caregivers' fingers when cleaning. Therefore, I developed two items for a mouth cleaning kit named "*Kyuty* [suction]" and "*Hotal* [firefly]." They are commercialized by Fine (https://www.fine-revolution.co.jp/). "*Kyuty*" is a type of toothbrush with a tube which is connected to a suction machine, so that you can clean the oral cavity while suctioning. Due to specific modifications on the tube and brush, we succeeded to make the suction power stronger than other similar brushes. "*Hotal*" is an example of an oral light tool which helps persons open their mouths. This kit helps caregivers to clean the oral cavity easily and speedily. Reduced bad breath was also reported by the nurses and caregivers after using this kit (Figure 6-10). You can learn how to use them on YouTube (https://www.youtube.com/watch?v=BZuwJsfQ9pk).

I have also created goods to prevent aspiration pneumonia: a small table over the bed that you can lower the height, a pillow to stop backward tilt-

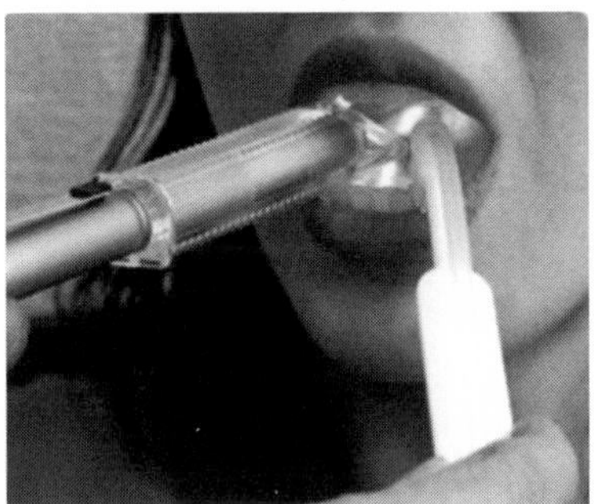

Figure 6-10 "*Kyuty*" and "*Hotal*"

ing, and a tray with tableware glued on to stop swallowing in one gulp. Users drink water/soup with a straw or spoon. Many persons with aspiration pneumonia tend to have dry mouth. I devised a mask with a special filter that moistens the oral cavity with a user's exhaled breath. See my website for more information (search with "Kiyoshi Yasuda homepage").

Recently, toothbrushes *"Possi"* by Kyocera & Lion allow users to hear music through bone conduction when he/she is attached with the teeth brush. Caregivers can take pictures of oral cavity by using *"NOVENINE SMASH"* by MOVENINE. Both of them may be used for persons who refuse toothbrushing or mouth opening (see Hickey & Bourgeois (2018) for eating and swallowing).

2.7 Summary of music therapy

Many studies have reported that the amount of cortisol, a stress hormone, decreases after listening to music (Nakajima, Ebihara, Saijo et al., 2013). This may be one explanation why music seems to be effective for behaviors of persons with dementia. Today, activities such as listening to music and singing songs are popular at many facilities as recreational activities. Some volunteer singers or music therapists might visit their homes, but it is difficult for them to visit the same person every day. Meanwhile, interventions introduced in this chapter can be carried out as many times as the person with dementia would like.

To my knowledge, this is the first demonstration that the automatic output of songs and messages succeeded to cope with challenging problems of persons with dementia at their homes (Mulvenna & Nugent, 2010). There are many persons who refuse to go to day-care, do not eat enough, or are easily agitated. The results of these studies indicate that the above interventions, or **the strategy of presenting information (music) in advance**, may be a successful method for managing persons with behavioral problems. In practical terms, this method holds great promise since it can easily be applied to other activities of daily life, such as bathing. I also created parodies (of songs) such as, "Let's go to the bathroom," "I can use eye drops," and "Let's brush teeth." Music is sometimes more effective than verbal persuasion for motivating persons with dementia and having them accomplish their daily tasks.

3. Communication support

Persons with dementia living at home tend to have little communication with their family members. Many of them still have the ability to enjoy having conversations, even as their dementia progresses. If they are given the opportunity to have conversations with the help of ATs when needed, it may be possible to reduce the frequency of challenging problems. In fact, the behaviors of persons with dementia are often alleviated after they start attending day-care centers and conversing with others there. Our experiment (Kuwahara, Yasuda, Tetsutani et al., 2010) also observed the reduction of challenging problems after they had opportunities for videophone conversations.

3.1 Assisting conversation using resources on websites

Some persons with dementia are unable to enjoy talking because they fail to recall keywords or topic-related memories of the past during conversation, even though they still have the ability to converse. We have released a vocabulary data file "*Rakuraku jiyuukaiwa* [easy and free conversation]" in a website (Yasuda et al., 2007b). It is a kind of dictionary in which words are categorized by topics to ensure easy access during conversation. This data file contains approximately 50,000 nouns and proper names which often become the keywords in conversation. For example, a list of famous mountains is useful when talking about mountain climbing. If you are a baseball fan, you can recall names of players by looking at a list of players' names (as of August 2021, the provider is repairing this site). Yasuda, Nemoto, Takenaka et al. (2007b) found that significantly more information was conveyed from persons with moderate/severe aphasia compared to other resources when the vocabulary data file was used (Figure 6-11). I asked a person with moderate dementia who was a former mountaineering enthusiast about what mountains he had climbed, but he could hardly remember

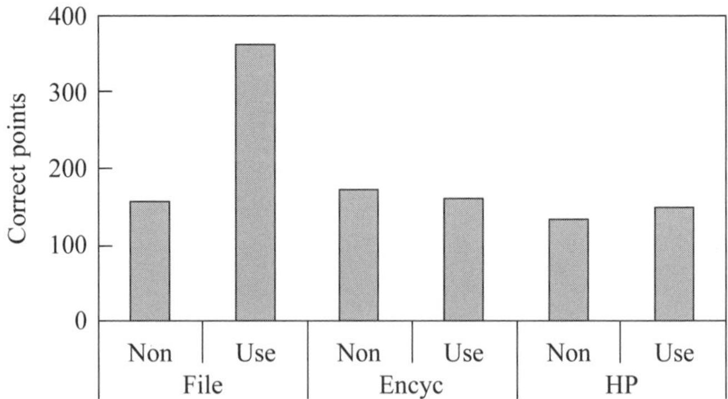

Figure 6-11 Total points in non-use and use conditions of three resources

Note: File = Vocabulary data file, Encyc = Encyclopedia, HP = Home page. Non, Use = The resource was not used, or used.

them. However, when I showed the list of 100 famous Japanese mountains in this file, he pointed to many mountains' names one after another.

Nakayama, Hara, & Nishio (2006) developed the *Wikipedia Thesaurus*, which is a system that can extract related keywords from the Wikipedia encyclopedia and exhibit them immediately after you input a search word. This system is useful as a keyword dictionary in various fields during conversations. Thus, by using the thesaurus, we can converse with a person with dementia who, for example, cannot recall a professional term in his former profession but still has preserved knowledge about it.

Currently, together with colleagues in the laboratory of Masao Fuketa at Tokushima University, we are developing the "*EDAHA*" system for activating conversation with persons with dementia. This system can exhibit related words, pictures and songs by a keyword on the monitor of PCs. If you input "New York" or "MLB (Major League Baseball)," for example, the system will show you related keywords and pictures, so that you can talk with a person with dementia who lived in New York, or liked baseball (Figure 6-12).

In the future, while showing keywords and pictures on the PC or tablet, a "*Mago* [grandchild] *agent*" (introduced in Section 2.1 of Chapter 7) will be able to ask questions to the user. For example, if the user was a farmer, the agent might ask technical questions such as the way to use pesticides appropriately. In most of the conversation systems developed so far, only simple conversation was possible which becomes boring before long. Be-

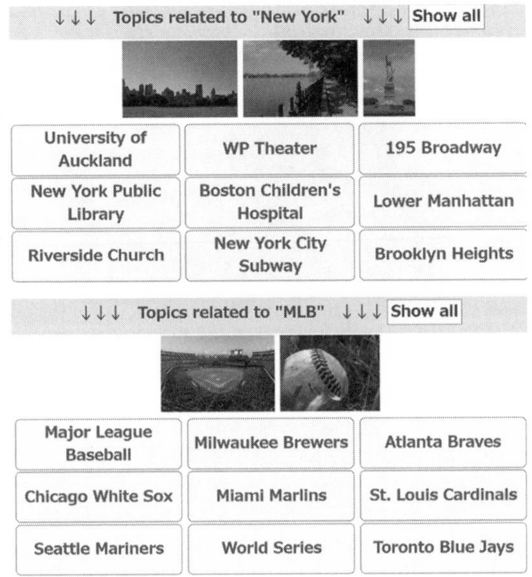

Figure 6-12 Exhibiting related words, pictures by "*EDAHA*" system

cause the voice recognition function at that time was still unstable, words of low frequency or professional terms seemed to be difficult to treat. On the other hand, our systems are based on the keywords presentation system and another type of conversation system. With our system, you will be able to have conversations with people in any professional field. We are trying to install the "*EDAHA*" system and the *mago* agent on tablet computers and on the robot "*Pepper*" by Softbank. You will also be able to use these systems on the videophone (see Section 2.2 in Chapter 7).

3.2 Conversation with volunteer companions on a videophone

Videophone is considered as one of the best communication tools for persons with dementia. Videophone conversation can reduce the depressed mood of the elderly. Furthermore, they can share various content such as written keywords, photos, movies, and music while they are conversing (Figure 6-13). Since 2003, I have been involved in a research project on supporting persons with dementia remotely by using a videophone at Advanced Telecommunications Research Institute International (ATR) (introduced in Chapter 7). The results of our experiments indicated that persons

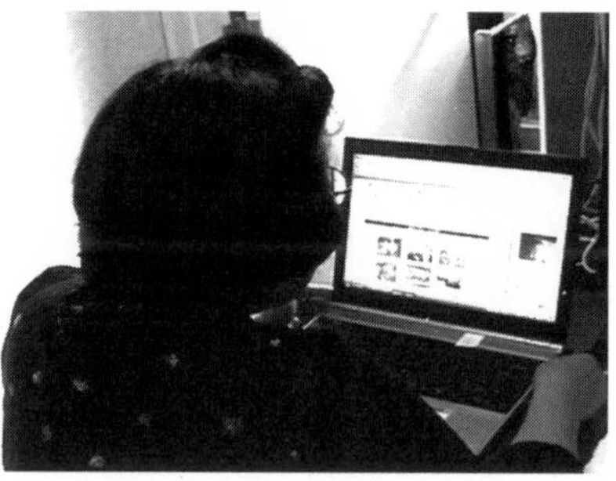

Figure 6-13 Videophone conversations between person with dementia and volunteer companion
Note: They are sharing related photos.

with dementia who had conversations on a videophone were more psychologically stable than those who watched TV programs (Kuwahara et al., 2010). A decrease of challenging problems was observed in some persons who had videophone conversation. It was also found that psychological stability of some persons lasted more than three hours after the conversation. Our second experiment also reported sustained psychological stability among the persons who had conversation on a videophone (Yasuda, Kuwahara, Kuwabara et al., 2013b).

The third follow-up study (Yasuda, Narumoto, Sano et al., 2019) also investigated the effectiveness of a videophone conversation for five participants with mild to moderate dementia (mean MMSE, 22.0). Two sessions were conducted. In Session A, participants conversed with a conversation companion through videophone for 30 min., and in Session B, participants watched their favorite TV programs for 30 min. Sessions A and B were rotated on a day-to-day basis. Their psychological stability immediately after each session was evaluated by family members using the revised GBS scale (Gottfries, Brane, Gullberg et al. (1982); concomitant evaluation) and the overall psychological stability three hours after each session (delayed evaluation) was also examined. Lower scores in the GBS scale mean better psychological stability (Figure 6-14). Significantly better psychological stability was obtained for two participants (Par. 3 and Par. 5) immediately (the concomitant evaluation), and one participant (Par. 3) three hours after the video conversation sessions (the delayed evaluation).

The common characteristic among persons in three studies (Kuwahara et al., 2010; Yasuda et al., 2013; 2019) who showed sustained stability was that they did not enjoy watching regular TV programs but they could still

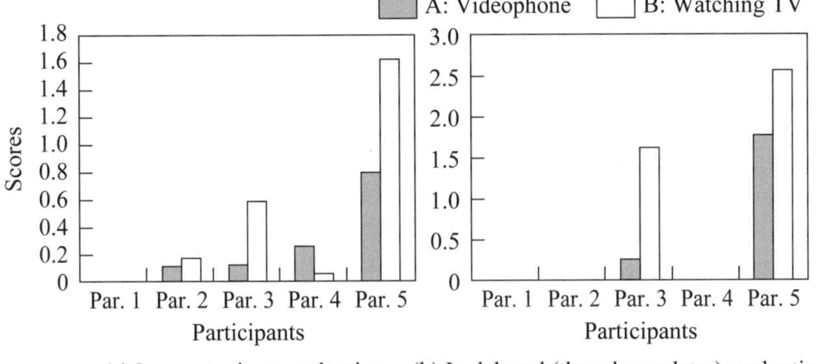

(a) In concomitant evaluation (b) In delayed (three hours later) evaluation

Figure 6-14 Average scores of five participants

Note: Par. = Participant; Lower score means psyhological stability.

enjoy having a conversation. This is an important clinical finding; it implies that if persons with dementia are given many opportunities to have conversations, responsive behaviors, such as the sundown syndrome, might not occur (Figure 6-14). We are expecting a follow-up study by other researchers.

While having conversations with persons with dementia, volunteer companions or others may face difficulties in searching for topics to talk about, since they often do not provide topics spontaneously. It is helpful to prepare reminiscence items such as old items or photos in advance, so that you can show them while conversing with the persons with dementia. You can also use the "*Rakuraku jiyuukaiwa*" website as described earlier. In addition, various kinds of videos or music can help you carry on your conversation. By "share screen", you can find photos and videos related to, for example, gardening on websites and talk about gardening while looking at them together. Showing items visually is beneficial especially for persons in the severe stage as they sometimes cannot communicate verbally.

Compared to normal face to face conversation, there are great advantages in using videophone conversation; you can talk about any topic with persons with dementia utilizing these digital contents. Today, you can use smartphone applications such as *LINE* to set up a videophone conversation and you could even have conversations in groups. If family members show their faces to persons remotely on their smartphones, it can give a sense of security to them, while family members can check their facial expressions (see Cheung & Peri (2021) for other information).

3.3 Launching a support group for videophone-conversation

Based on the results described above and with the support from the laboratory of Noriaki Kuwahara at Kyoto Institute of Technology, we launched a "support group for videophone-conversation" in November, 2015. Currently, seven volunteer conversation companions have a 30-minute conversation with each of six persons with dementia 2 to 4 times a month. In order to start up a videophone conversation, volunteers for PC operation in our group visited the persons' homes, installed the free videophone software "*Skype*," and instructed the persons and family members on how to use the system. In this way, they began having conversations with volunteer companions. Currently, you can use our service free of charge. Recently, our cooperative volunteer organizations "*Hidamari*" and "*Ichihara Silver College 21*" started providing remote conversation companions and music therapy to residents in elderly facilities.

We can also utilize "**an automatic response function at incoming calls**" on Skype. With this function, users do not need to operate the device as long as the switch is on (in the sleep mode). Conversations can be started with a call by a volunteer companion. That is, what the person with dementia has to do is to wait for an incoming call from the companion. Once the system is set up, it can also be used by family members as a remote surveillance system for them. If they can build a network not only with volunteer companions but also with children, grandchildren, friends of persons, medical/care professionals, and if persons with dementia can have a conversation with those people on a daily rotation, the family members may be able to reduce the frequency of challenging problems.

DFJI-Zoom café has been holding a group conversation between persons with dementia and family members/supporters once a month since 2017 (http://www.dementia-friendly-japan.jp/). The Café Le Brain by the Dementia Alliance International (DAI) is a monthly online café, where members can enjoy discussion and receive support (https://www.dementiaallianceinternational.org/events/cafe-le-brain/). The Board meeting also provide members with update information prior to this online café. The online cafés are open to people with dementia and their families, friends or care partners who support them.

Today, the effects of remote support using videophone have been reported by several family members on websites such as "*Remote care from a 40-year-old* (http://40kaigo.net/).” Private companies have also started a paid service for videophone conversation. A remote-care service called “*Mimamorin* [surveillance]” by Exceliebe provides such a service for 10 to 80 dollars a month (a 5 to 30 minute conversation once a week). Another conversation service “*Yunaito call*” by Est is for residents in care facilities. The “*Joyce* videophone” by My Joice is a system in which conversation is made possible by connecting the Internet and a camera to an ordinary TV (at 60 dollars a month).

3.4 A global network of videophones among persons with dementia

As the number of persons with dementia is undoubtedly on the increase, volunteer conversation companions will be scarce in the future, even if a remote network is set up. Meanwhile, as persons with moderate and severe dementia talk about the same topics repeatedly every time, it may cause stress on some healthy conversation companions. One of the ways to solve this problem is to let persons with mild dementia converse with other persons with dementia (Yasuda, 2008). Even if they talk about the same topics over again, the talking partners who also have dementia are likely to have forgotten the content of the previous sessions. In this case, the talking partners are less likely to feel stress compared to the healthy volunteer companions.

Some persons with early-onset dementia say that, “We still want to be helpful to society.” They are advised to become a volunteer companion for those who have the same disease. Alarms should be set to notify them of the scheduled conversations. Conversation topics should be prepared in advance. Books of autobiographical information and reminiscence related topics may be useful for volunteer companions to ask relevant questions. Such volunteer work might become a job for persons with early-onset dementia in the future. When the stage of dementia progresses to moderate and severe dementia, those persons might be helped by other companions with mild dementia. I call this mutual support-help relation the “*Ninnin* [dementia-dementia]” supporting system, in which a person with dementia has to take care of another person with dementia (Yasuda, 2008a). Engineers are expected to develop interfaces by which persons with dementia or volunteer companions are reminded of the schedule for conversation and can get started with a minimal amount of preparation for suitable topic lists for each person.

Persons with dementia sometimes feel restless at night. If they can talk with companions on the videophone, it might be greatly helpful for the persons and family members. It is not easy, however, to find a volunteer companions who can talk to them at midnight. In such a case, Japanese speakers living overseas could be helpful by taking advantage of time differences. For example, many people who speak Japanese live in Brazil, which has a 12-hour time difference. They may happily help persons with dementia in Japan with conversations (Yasuda, 2008a).

In 2011, when I had a chance to visit Paris, I asked a Japanese association in Paris to search for volunteers for conversation companions for persons with dementia in Japan. Some of the Japanese people in the association said that they had left their parents of old age in Japan and were worried about their health, including dementia. Furthermore, if foreign students who are learning the Japanese language have opportunities to talk with persons with dementia, they can become Japanese teachers for them. Hearing the same questions that the persons with dementia repeatedly ask and making comments may be a good way to study the language. This international assistance system could be applied in many countries.

According to WHO, the number of persons with dementia will be over 100 million in the world after a few decades. I hope that people will recycle their used/old smartphones, tablets, and PCs to the persons with dementia in the world, so that they can have the means to have conversations regardless of time, place, and financial means. Fortunately, translation technologies between different languages are improving rapidly. It is possible, for example, that a Japanese person with dementia will be able to ask a Russian for advice by using a translation application. In this way, global support networks for conversation will be built. In the near future, various remote support systems, not limited to conversation, will be possible by using networks for persons with dementia and their family members.

CHAPTER SEVEN

Research on daily life support using agents and other advanced technologies

Since the beginning of the 21st century, research using Information-Communication-Technology (ICT) has evaluated supportive technology for the daily life of persons with dementia. Currently, Artificial Intelligence (AI) technology is being applied in various fields and its impacts on the social life of people are being discussed. I suggested the following points to researchers at the conference of the Japanese Society for Artificial Intelligence in 2012; "Artificial prosthetic joints or artificial hearts have been developed for patients whose joints or hearts are dysfunctional. In a similar sense, artificial intelligence should be utilized preferentially for persons whose intelligence or memory is deficient due to brain impairments or other diseases." Similar to the creation of barrier-free space in physical environments, intelligence- and memory-free society should also be created. For example in Chapter 5, a "Memory Sharing" system was introduced. In a similar way, if smartglasses are worn, "AI secretary" or remote friends will help persons judge situations and take the appropriate actions. AI has the potential to make life comfortable for both persons with dementia and the healthy elderly.

In this chapter, the history of High-Tech AT will be reviewed briefly in the first section, and then current trials using High-Tech AT for persons with dementia will be described in the second section. Some of the High-Tech AT are expected to be applied in our daily lives in the coming years and should become as practical as Middle-Tech AT. In the third section, the new concept of "dementia-assistance dog" will be proposed. See the reviews of Bateman, Srinivas, Emmett et al. (2017); Meiland, Innes, Mountain et al. (2017); Ienca, Fabrice, Elger et al. (2017) for other research studies conducted on daily life support with High-Tech AT.

1. The history of High-Tech AT for dementia

Around the year 2000, the BIME research center in the U.K. began a project on AT-development for persons with dementia. Other projects also started in Europe, such as ASTRAID, Enable, and Independent. Some examples of the AT developed by these projects are a device that displays elapsed time, an electric calendar that differentiates morning and afternoon, a cabinet with hidden locks, a remote controller with a limited selection of buttons, a CD player and a radio with one button, and telephones with which you make a call by pressing photos of a person's face. Smart houses built by Dementia VoICe and BIME were equipped with AT to deal with problems which were common among persons with dementia. The AT installed in the house included a voice alarm to stop them from going out, directional guidance by sequentially turning on and off lights in the corridor, a temperature sensor to prevent burning pots while cooking, and a surveillance system for lost belongings. Similar research was also conducted in other institutions such as the University of Dundee, the University of Toronto, and Georgia Institute of Technology (see Astell et al. (2019) in the references).

In 2003, the ATR's Intelligent Robotics and Communication Laboratories in Japan started a project called "Information therapy projects" for supporting persons with dementia. I took part in the project from the beginning. The first project focused on remote support for persons by using a videophone and other advanced technologies, since the remote assistance was a promising and unexplored discipline at that time. The ATs studied in the project were as follows: automatic displays of the daily schedule, automatic output of favorite music and videos for each person, simple interfaces by which they can have a conversation on a videophone, an *anime* agent with which they can talk, and an assistance system for elimination by monitoring each step of toileting procedures (Kuwahara, Kuwabara, Utsumi et al., 2004; Kuwahara, Kuwabara, Tetsutani et al., 2005). Three studies will be described from the project in the following sections.

1.1 Automatically changing of TV programs

As seen in Chapter 6, the number of TV programs or scenes that persons with moderate/severe dementia enjoy are decreasing. Furthermore, it also becomes difficult for them to select favorite programs and to operate the remote controller. Usually, when the program is not interesting to us, we turn our face away from the TV. In the content-switching system (Kawato, Utsumi, & Abe, 2006), facial orientation was detected by an infrared camera. Then, the watcher's attention to the displayed contents was estimated. If the estimated attention level was low, the content was changed automatically to another program. If family members recorded only scenes in which persons showed their interest, a customized video collection could be provided. Recently, as the real-time recognition of gaze and facial expression is becoming possible, a more accurate system can be created.

1.2 Accomplishment of daily tasks through watching videos

Assistance in the execution of daily tasks through the Sony IC Recorder (ICD-PX240; IC Rec) has already been introduced in Chapter 3. The verbal messages by the IC Rec, however, were ineffective for some persons with dementia. With the expectation of higher probability to achieve daily tasks, Kuwahara, Yasuda, Tetsutani et al. (2010) developed a video and schedule prompter system. Four persons participated in the study. In order for the persons with dementia to accomplish daily tasks, such as taking medicines, doing exercise, keeping a diary, and others, more than 10 kinds of task-promoting videos were created. Then, one of the videos that each person with dementia selected was set to play automatically on the person's personal computer. The same procedures were executed for the remaining three persons. At the beginning of each video, one of the research members appeared on the monitor and explained the importance of doing the task and asked the person to carry out the task, which each person had promised to do. The results showed that the average achievement ratio for the tasks of four persons was 52 %, which we considered to be insufficient achievement. It appeared that persons with dementia tended to lose their motivation to do the daily tasks.

In our past experiments (Chapter 6), however, automatic output of music and personalized reminiscence photo videos improved their behaviors and concentration levels. Based on these results, it was hypothesized that if the reminiscence photo videos were played preceding the task-promoting videos, their achievement ratio would increase. Therefore, the reminiscence photo videos were presented to four other participants with dementia for about ten minutes ahead of each task-promoting video in the ABBA design experiment (Yasuda, Kuwahara, Kuwabara et al., 2013b). As expected, the average achievement ratio for the daily tasks by the four participants went

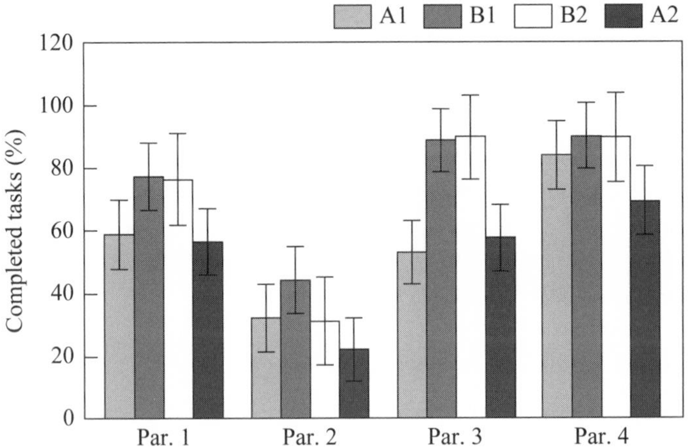

Figure 7-1 Average percentages of scheduled completed tasks
Notes: A1 and A2 = family members' instruction. B1 and B2 = task-promoting and reminiscence photo videos. Par. = participant.

up significantly to 82 % (B1 and B2 in Figure 7-1). Therefore, the importance of motivating persons with dementia prior to giving instructions was confirmed.

This system can also automatically record persons' behaviors at set times. For example, when they are asked to take medicines, their family members can check the recording later on by the Internet. Today, it is possible to play videos automatically by using digital photo frames and application programs on a smartphone (as described in Chapters 5 and 6). These functions should be utilized more in assisting persons with dementia.

1.3 Procedures for assisting with toileting

As the stage of dementia becomes more severe, persons may fail to accomplish elimination procedures in the toilet. Consequently, they soil their underwear, the inside of the toilet, and even the corridors. These failures increase the burden of their family members. Utsumi, Kanbara, Kawato et al. (2006) developed a system to assist persons with dementia in carrying out elimination procedures by using infra-red dot patterns in the toilet. With this system, the posture of each action by the person was recognized through "blurred" images, which was to protect their privacy (Figure 7-2). If they failed to take an appropriate action, such as flushing the toilet or using toilet paper, verbal instructions and sample animation videos were

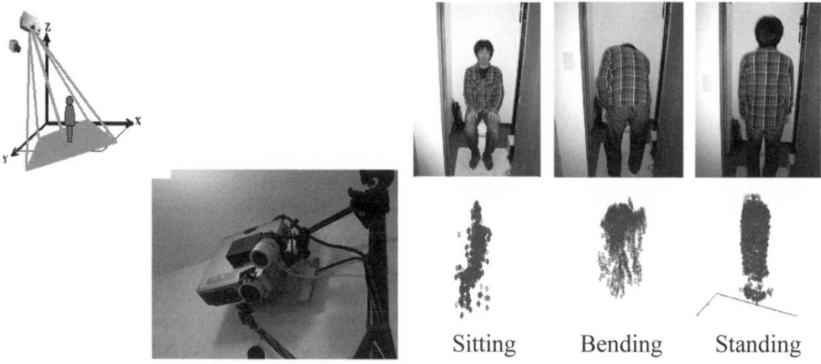

Figure 7-2 System for toileting assistance

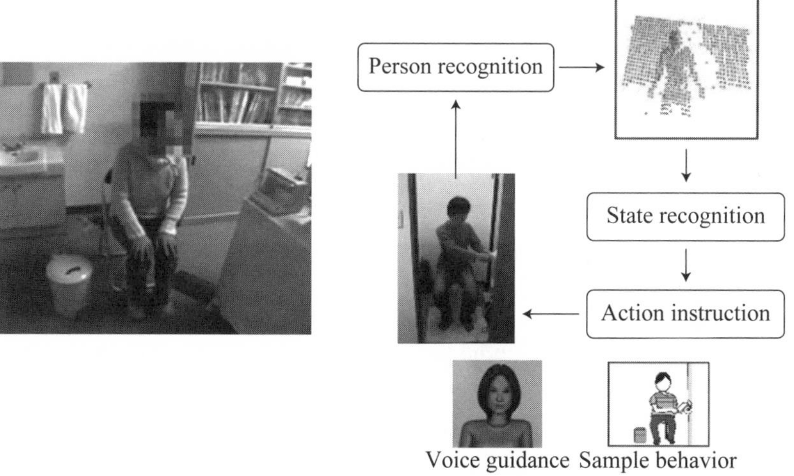

Figure 7-3 Preliminary experiment in simulated toilet environment

given through a personal computer set on the toilet wall (Figure 7-3). In this way, necessary actions were monitored step by step and advice for each action was given sequentially when needed. As far as we know, this was the first system to assist persons with dementia in performing their toileting behaviors.

Yasuda, Okazaki, Utsumi et al. (2008c) conducted a preliminary experiment with seven participants with mild to severe dementia (range of MMSE was 8–28, mean = 21.5) in a simulated toilet environment. The participants were not informed of the purpose of the study. The experimenter told each of them, "Please, follow the instructions on the computer after you enter the room." They were required to perform nine sequential actions, step by step. The required actions were the simulated actions such as touch your knees (pull down your pants), take a sheet of paper, throw the paper into a box, press a button (flush water), etc. The positions of the paper, boxes, and button were automatically identified with an LED lamp and buzzer at the step when each is needed. If it was automatically determined that the person performed an out of sequence action, the previous action was instructed again. The examiner watched them with a camera in the next room.

A favorable result was gained from the experiment; 5 out of 7 participants were able to perform the nine sequential actions according to the instructions given by the animation videos (Figure 7-3). One of the two participants who could not complete the required actions had the most severe dementia (MMSE score, 8). When she was instructed to take the sheet of paper from the box next to the monitor, she could not move her gaze to the box. Instead, she tried to take the sample *anime* paper on the screen. In this situation we should have erased the image on screen.

2. Current High-Tech AT research for dementia

2.1 Conversations with anime agents

We suggested in Chapter 6 that the psychological stability of persons with dementia may last for three hours after having a conversation on a videophone. If that is the case, we should set up a system in which they are able to talk with volunteer companions 24 hours a day, since some persons with dementia might want to have a conversation even in the night. It is truly difficult, however, to launch such a system immediately in which they can converse with companions at any time.

As a solution to this problem, we developed an *anime* agent system whereby persons can have conversations with the agent on a computer screen. The system was developed together with colleagues at the laboratory of Yukiko Nakano at Seikei University. In this system, the *anime* agent asks questions such as, "Have you slept well?" or "How is your physical condition?" Users are expected to respond verbally in a fixed time. If the system cannot detect their voice any more in the fixed time, the response is regarded as finished. The *anime* agent will then move on to ask the next question (Sakai, Nonaka, Yasuda et al., 2012). Our experience revealed that an interval of 3.5 seconds is the appropriate fixed time for pauses between questions, although the fixed time can be modified for each person. The preliminary experiments suggest that if the questions are interesting for the person, he/she continues the conversation with the agent by responding verbally. This means that interactive conversations with agents are possible by detecting any verbal response, without needing to use speech recognition systems which are popular but often unstable in recognizing speech in real circumstances.

Based on the above results, we developed a system called "*Anime mago* [grandchild] *agent reminiscence conversation system*" in collaboration with the Institute of Language Understanding Inc. and the laboratory of Junichi Aoe at Tokushima University. With this system, the "grandchild agent" on a computer screen asks reminiscence questions to a person (Figure 7-4). The questions prepared were 120 (now 450) in total and they were categorized into eight groups such as school, hobby, job, health, etc. In this system, the interval of 3.5 seconds was set as an initial fixed time for responding.

In a trial, one participant told us about his impression of the first version of this system as follows: "The continuous questioning to me was like a police interrogation." Therefore, in the second version and thereafter, we attached anecdotes spoken by the agent before each question. The *anime* agent told a short story about his own experiences, traditional customs, etc. Then, he asked the participant questions on the same topic of his anecdote (Table 7-1).

The second version succeeded in eliciting positive reactions from participants. Some participants began crying with happiness after a 30 minute conversation with the agent. A man with early-onset dementia began singing along with the agent and said, "I want to go home with this child and

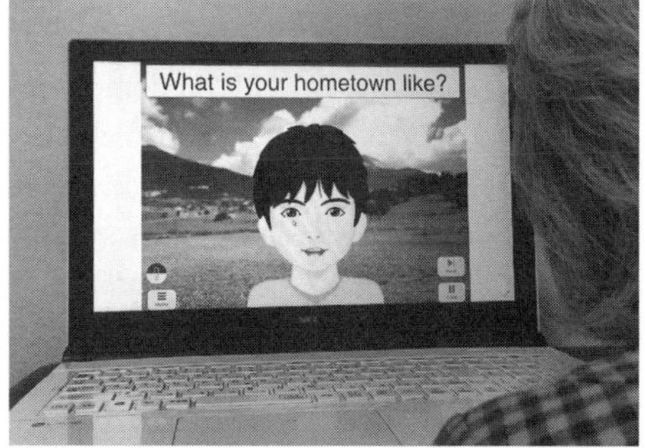

Figure 7-4 "*Mago* [grandchild] *agent reminiscence conversation system*"

Table 7-1 Example of questions by *anime* agent

Anecdotes spoken by agent	Questions for user
I like movies with robots on TV.	*What kind of movies did you watch when you were young?*
I've never been on an airplane before. I'd like to go to a foreign country by plane.	*Have you ever taken an airplane to a faraway place?*
In March, my aunt had a wedding at a hotel in Tokyo. There were a lot of people there and it was very lively.	*Did you have a wedding? If so, what was your wedding like?*
My grandfather's blood pressure is high, so the doctor told him to avoid salty foods.	*Do you have high blood pressure? Or do you avoid salty foods?*

talk with him at home." Most of the other agent conversation systems at that time focused on how to reply to utterances from users based on speech recognition systems. The focus of our system is, however, different from theirs. Our focus is to tap the memories that users still have and to encourage them to talk as long as they want. In fact, some persons continued talking with the agent over one hour. Excessive engagement in this talking system, however, may cause unexpected side effects such as overexcitement, forgetting to go to the toilet, etc. Consequently, a function was added to stop the system automatically at a set time in the third version. When the end time approaches, the agent says, "Now, I have to do my homework. Bye!"

The *anime* agent asked reminiscence questions to eight participants with dementia in the experiment using the third version. Meanwhile, an adult companion (one of the authors) also asked the same questions to the same participants on other days. The total number of mora (Japanese syllables) spoken with the agent was 5,494 (74 %) compared to 7,406 (100 %) with the companion (Figure 7-5) (Yasuda, Aoe, & Fuketa, 2013).

This system might be more practical if the conversation is conducted in a quiet room. The system has a function to make it start at set times automatically. Thus, it is very helpful for persons with challenging problems such as sundowning. If they are focused on conversing with the agent, they may forget that they wanted to go to their "old house." Currently, researchers at the laboratory of Masao Fuketa at Tokushima University and the Institute of Language Understanding Inc. are developing a newer version of the system to be used on tablets and smartphones as well as foreign lan-

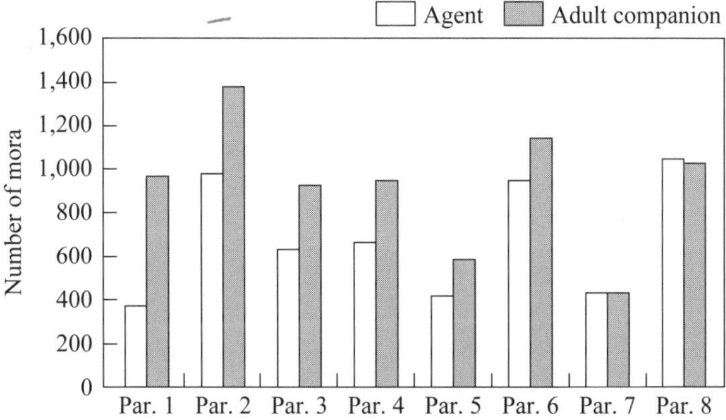

Figure 7-5 Number of mora in 8 participants' replies

Note: Par. = participant.

guage versions. This system, as well as the "*EDAHA*" mentioned in Section 3.1 of Chapter 6, are also planned to be installed in the robot "*Pepper*" by Softbank. Pepper is movable and equipped with a big monitor on its chest. Pepper will automatically approach users and start reminiscence conversations with them in the near future.

2.2 Anime agent as a facilitator during group conversations

For persons with dementia, conversation is extremely important for their psychological stability as discussed previously. While volunteer conversation companions may be limited, the number of persons with dementia

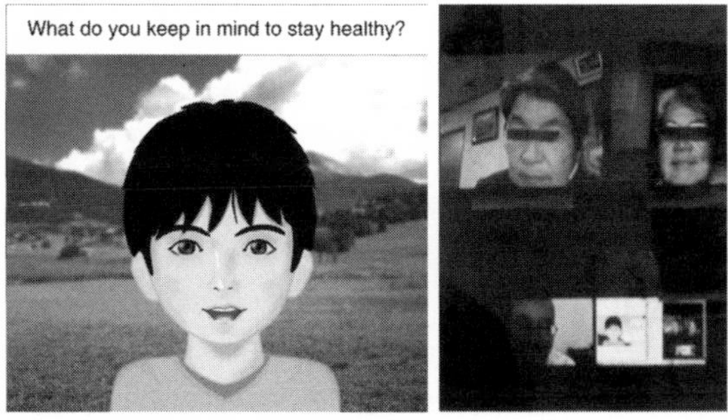

Figure 7-6 Conversation among two persons with dementia and *anime* agent

Source: Recreated by the author based on Yasuda et al. (2016b).

will be increasing. Accordingly, a remote group conversation among them is needed, but a shortage of facilitators is anticipated. Therefore, Yasuda, Fuketa, Morita et al. (2016b) conducted an experiment with Skype in which the *anime* agent acted as a facilitator for a remote conversation held by two persons with moderate dementia (Figure 7-6). The interval of six seconds was set as an initial fixed time for the agent to respond. If chatting did not occur between them in the six-second fixed interval, the *anime* agent automatically provided the next topic. The first author participated as an observer. Meanwhile, a human facilitator also had a conversation with the same persons and talked about the same topics on another day.

The quality of two recorded conversations was later assessed independently by three evaluators. They evaluated the quality of each conversation on a 1-5 point psychological scale. The average of their evaluation for the conversation chaired by the *anime* agent was the mean of 3.9 compared with that of the human facilitator (4.9) (Yasuda et al., 2016b). This *anime* agent system is, therefore, considered to be practical for group conversations by persons with dementia.

Related Topics —An agent system for persons who have lost speech or memory—
The most severe level of aphasia is called "global aphasia." Persons with this level have severe impairments not only in understanding language but also speaking, writing, and expressing in gesture. In 1998, when cellphones became popular, I thought of an agent system by which even persons with global aphasia can "speak." At first you upload detailed data about a user with aphasia on a storage center of the Internet, and when the user has a conversation, she/he holds out her/his cellphone to the other person and then lets the person ask questions to the phone. When asked, the agent will reply automatically to the person on behalf of the user with aphasia from the accumulated data on the Internet. The conversation could be, for example, "Where are you from?" Then, the agent replies, "I am from Kamogawa in Chiba." This is a "communication agent" system by utilizing advanced technology for speech.

Now by using smartphones it may be possible for persons with aphasia even to ask "voluntarily" to another person based on conversation records as well as recognition of the faces. This system could also be used as a "memory agent" for persons with severe dementia who have begun losing their own episodic memories. In the last 20 years, face and speech recognition technology has made dramatic progress, and thus I hope that engineering researchers will develop this kind of alternative agent systems. In the meantime, elderly people should start entering their daily events and biographical data into their smartphone or PC, preparing for the possibility of having severe aphasia or dementia. The data will be utilized for your "communication" or "memory" agent.

2.3 Communications with persons who use stereotypical utterances

When dementia is at a profound stage, persons have difficulties understanding and speaking sentences, and even words. At this stage, some of them roar, mutter to themselves, make babbling noises and use stereotypical words. It is considered to be difficult for family members and staff members of facilities to have verbal conversations with them, and instead non-verbal communication, such as touch and gestures, is recommended. I once met a bedridden person with severe dementia. She was muttering to herself with unintelligible jargon. I tried returning the same jargon to her that she just said. After several minutes she suddenly said, "*Arigato* [thank you]". Thus, persons at this stage of dementia may still have a desire to interact verbally with others, but new approaches to communication should be considered.

Oshima, Itou, Nishimoto et al. (2013) in the laboratory of Koichi Nakayama at Saga University proposed an interaction system in which utterances of persons with dementia are transformed musically through two microphones and then played back to them. By this verbal-musical interaction system, their utterances are transformed into the sol-fa pitch (e.g., do, re, mi) in real time. Then, they are played back musical phrases (consisting of

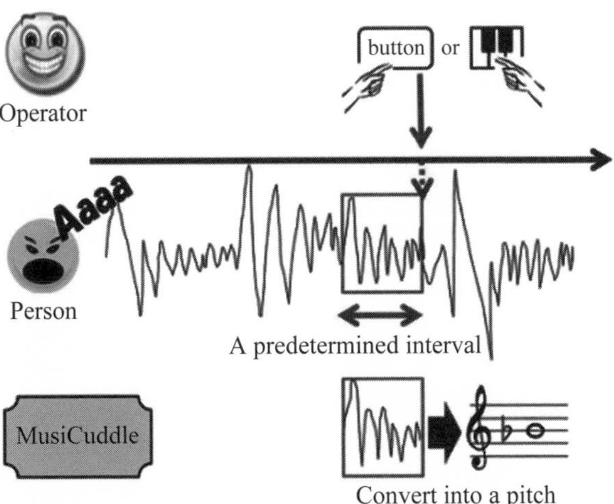

Figure 7-7 MusiCuddle; verbal-musical interaction system

very short phrases lasting 3–30 seconds). The phrase starts with a pitch and rhythm that matches their utterance and estimated mood (Figure 7-7). By repeating this interaction, verbal communication will be possible although it is based on the prosody of the utterance that reflects emotional states. Although this experiment is very preliminary, we should continue to search for new ways to communicate with persons with profound dementia.

2.4 Assisting system for cooking

Cooking is one of the most important activities of our lives. It is not only connected with the joy of eating but also deeply relates to health, entertainment, and communication. Since cooking requires various procedures, it becomes hard work for persons with cognitive impairments. Sano, Miyawaki, Mitsumori et al. (2013) proposed a cooking navigation system that consists of static and dynamic cooking recipes. During the cooking process, a number of tasks are generally done simultaneously. For example, a total of 20 steps are required to make simmered meat and potatoes. They arranged a PC screen with a video section at the left side and a comment section at the right side. When a user clicks on the screen, a short video is played for the next procedure. Comments like, "You worked well!" or cautionary notes like, "You have to glance at the pan!" are also emitted. The FOOD (Framework for optimizing the process of feeding) project aims at building a "smart" kitchen environment, providing older adults with services supporting safety, motivation and fun in the kitchen, and a healthy lifestyle (Grossi, Bianchi, Matrella et al., 2014). More research studies are expected to be conducted to support the procedural tasks of their daily lives.

2.5 Compensatory system for outings

Today, images of most streets and the surrounding scenery in the world can be seen by using websites such as, "Google street view" by Google. With this app you can virtually "walk" anywhere in the world while staying at home. We are developing a "walking" system collaborating with Yutaka Takase in the laboratory of Yukiko Nakano at Seikei University (Takase, Yoshida, Dohi et al., 2016). With this system, when persons with dementia wish to go, for example, to their parent's home, you show them the streets near the home on the screen. If they move their legs in front of the screen on which the images of the streets are projected, they can walk on the images of the streets which move according to their steps (Figure 7-8).

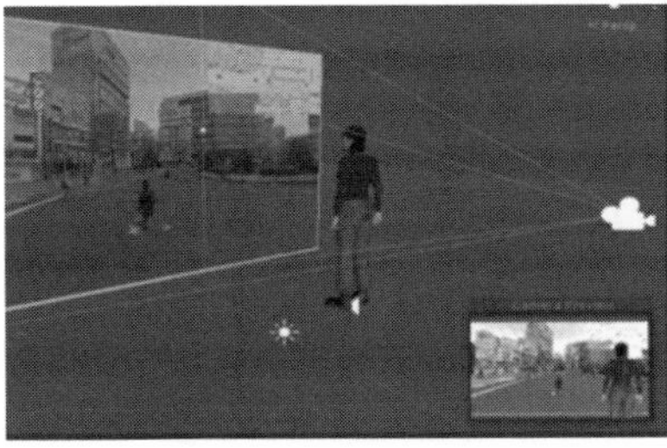

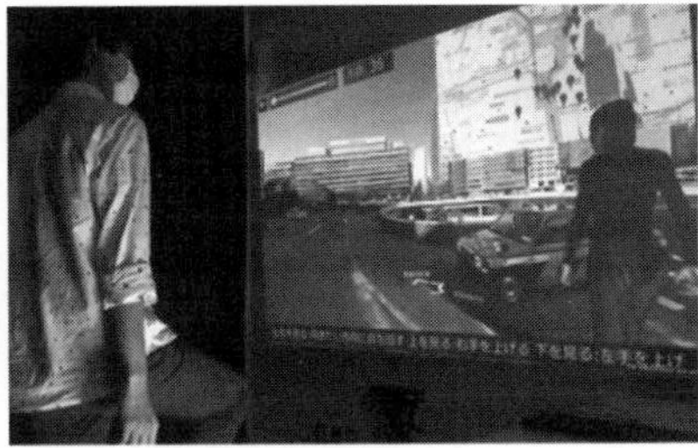

Figure 7-8 Compensatory system for outings

In addition, an *anime* agent appears on the screen and acts as a guide for the person with dementia. The *anime* agent will escort him/her on the screen and take him/her to the destination while conversing with the person and explaining about the surrounding scenery. In this intervention, persons with dementia can have reminiscence conversations, as well as practice walking in a familiar location. This system allows persons with dementia to safely visit wherever they what to go, for example, to the summit of Mount *Fuji* or even to the moon, while staying in their rooms. This compensatory system for outings should be studied more for practical use by persons with dementia who want to go back to their "old homes." Engineers are expected to recreate old images of streets/scenery that no longer exist. Persons may feel comforted by the images of past locations instead of present images of locations that are not familiar.

2.6 A "smart" support system with anime agents in homes

Today, many surveillance systems are available on the market for overseeing persons with dementia in their rooms, but many of them are one-way systems which lack mutual interactions. Recently, some systems have begun to have a function with which persons can have videophone conversations with remote family members. Yet, there have been no studies asking persons about their plans, feelings, forgetfulness, or concerns they might have at any particular time. The principle of person centered-care should also be realized for this advanced technology by asking their opinion.

Together with researchers at the laboratory of Masahide Nakamura of Kobe University, we are developing a system whereby an *anime* agent in a person's PC asks the person about the present physical or mental situations. Sensors set at several locations in the person's home can detect any changes in the light, temperature, vibration, and so forth. Immediately after any

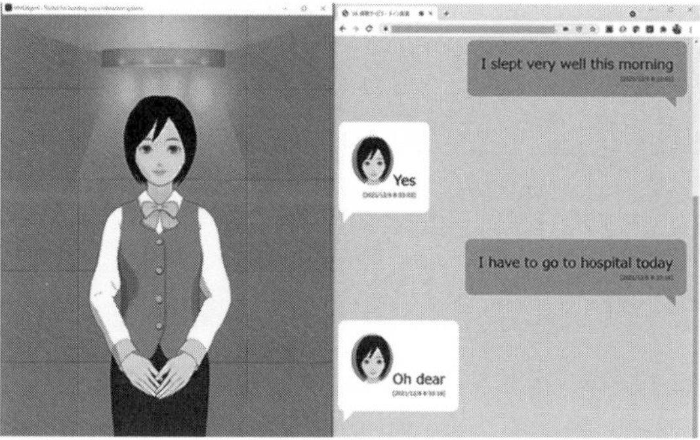

Figure 7-9 Smart support system with *anime* agent

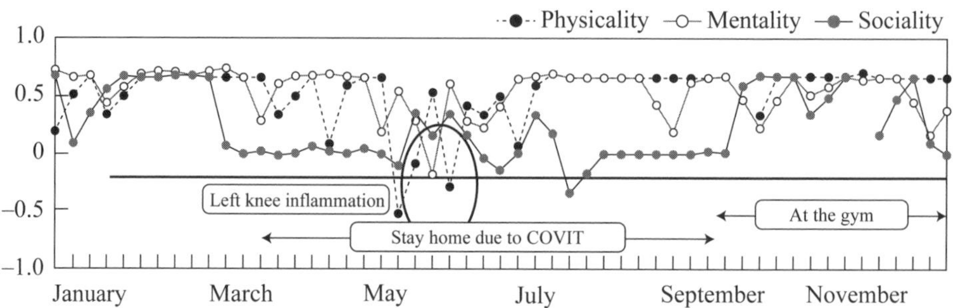

Figure 7-10 Result of self-reported conditions by a man in his seventies

Notes: The low sociability from March to October in 2020 was the result of the home-evacuation from the Covid-19. It has improved since he started going to the gym again in November. Inflammation of his right knee worsened from mid-May to mid-July. His physicality and mentality also deteriorated in this period.

changes are detected, the agent asks the person what happened (Tokunaga, Tamamizu, Saiki et al., 2016; Tamamizu, Sakakibara, Saiki et al., 2017). For example, when a light was switched on in the morning, the agent asks, "It seems that you got up now. Did you sleep well?" (Figure 7-9). Without asking immediately, the person with dementia may easily forget the things that happened. The agent can also ask the person at specific set times, for example, "What did you eat for lunch?" in the afternoon. Further, we prepared seven questions about physicality, mentality, sociality, etc. Then, one of them is asked regularly every week (Miura, Saiki, Nakamura et al, 2021) (Figure 7-10). Persons with dementia can also voluntarily enter utterances by just clicking a big icon on the screen whenever they want.

These questions are also delivered to persons' and family members' smartphones, so the persons can enter utterances as well as photos and auditory recordings anywhere outside their home. The family member can also enter correct or supplemental information. When the users open the PC, a list of utterances entered the day before appears. They are advised to correct manually inaccurate information of the utterances. In this process, they can confirm what they have done, or the information provided by the family members, such as answers to their questions.

Persons with MCI/dementia can search for the entered utterances, photos and recordings by date and times as well as keywords on their PC. If they entered, "I put my wallet in the top drawer", or a photo of the wallet, they can access these data with the keyword "Wallet". Further, if they classify each item of data into categories on their PC, category-based searching is also possible (Maeda, Saiki, Nakamura et al., 2019). For example, if they open the category of "forgetfulness," they can see the list of forgotten episodes of the past (Figure 7-11). They can remember what and how many times they have forgotten. This system is being tested out at several homes since 2016 (Tamamizu et al., 2017). In the near future, the agent will suggest appropriate coping strategies or memory aids to them.

When the room temperature is too high, the agent asks, "Aren't you hot? Would you like to turn on your air conditioner?" If the person agrees, the air conditioner and other home appliances can be switched on by using IoT

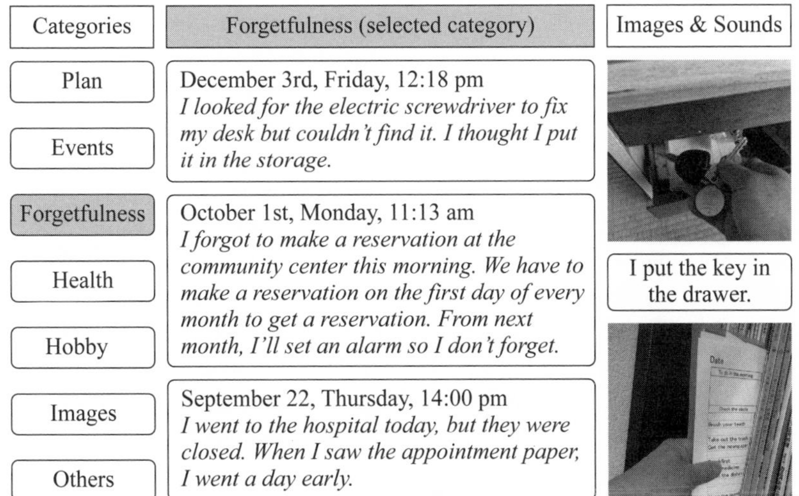

Figure 7-11 List of forgotten episodes of the past

(Internet of Things) technology. We also aim to create a system for when they say, "I am not motivated to do anything," a list of musical selections would appear from which they could make a selection. When they say, "I feel lonely," photos of the grandchildren could be shown, and they would be able to decide to chat with the grandchildren on videophone. To increase their motivation, the agent's face and expression can be changed to the face of a preferred person (Nakatani, Saiki, Nakamura et al., 2018).

We are also planning to have the agent do more tasks, such as to set schedules, to search for something on the Internet, to provide video programs (e.g., gymnastics, quizzes), to open a 24-hour videophone chat room, to emit verbal messages via speakers at key points in the house (e.g., flush water in the toilet) (Ozono, Chen, Nakamura et al., 2021). I have been inputting biometric information verbally such as blood pressure, sleep time, etc. into this system for the past several years. Currently, the agent system can automatically incorporate such data by wearing a smartwatch. If one of the numerical values exceeds the healthy threshold, the agent will notify and advise the user to take appropriate coping strategies.

2.7 Smartglasses and augmented/mixed reality

Wearers can see or get various information by wearing smartglasses. "*FRAMES ALTO*" by BOSE are a sunglasses-type wireless earphone. It is comfortable to wear and does not block the ear canal. In collaboration with a smartphone, you can listen to music while walking, and receive voice guidance from the google map. The weather and other information can also be checked. You can call your family through Siri App.

Another version of smartglasses allows users to send information about the situation in front of them to their remote family members by using the camera attached to the glasses, and then receiving instructions back from the family members. For example, the wearer of smartglasses sends the video of a broken machine to a remote instructor to receive repair guidance. "*Ray-Ban Stories*" by Facebook & EssilorLuxottica allow users to take and store hundreds of photos or dozens of videos on the glasses before transferring to their smartphones via an app. The weight of the glasses is less than 50 grams. The battery life is advertised as "all-day." An LED lump will glow to indicate to the people around that a video is being recorded by the user.

Smartglasses like "*MOVERIO*" by Epson are translucent glasses on to which the screen images of a personal computer can be projected. You can see the things in front of you while also seeing the projected information.

Schedules, instructions from family members, and manuals on how to use devices can be projected onto the lenses. Today, it is possible to project onto the glasses the names of persons, objects, and places that users are currently observing. This system is called the overlay of "augmented reality" or "mixed reality (MR)." I had some persons with dementia who wore smartglasses and read projected images on the glasses. None of them reported any discomfort. It will be a very useful AT especially for persons with MCI and early-onset dementia who are still at work. Today, smartglasses come in a variety of styles, such as a one-glass version with which you can turn the small display to the front of your eye as necessary (Figure 7-12).

When dementia progresses to the middle or severe stage, persons may feel uncomfortable in their own environments; they may not recognize familiar streets and the scenery around them. This may be because they have episodic memory deficits. The systems mentioned above will have the capability to superimpose digital images onto a field of view which allows the wearer to see more comfortable surroundings. Evaluations of smartglasses for assisting the elderly are underway (see Blattgerste, Renner, & Pfeiffer (2019) and Ferreira, Ferreira, Cavaco et al. (2020)).

A person with Alzheimer's disease who was an accountant started folding pages of magazines and newspapers repeatedly every day as if he was working in the office. In order to have the person devote himself to his "work" comfortably, his previous "work place" could be projected onto the surrounding walls or curtains. Abe (2017) demonstrated that if a person's face and body are projected onto a semi-circle-shaped screen, the person appears three-dimensionally. If this method is used, he may be able to work

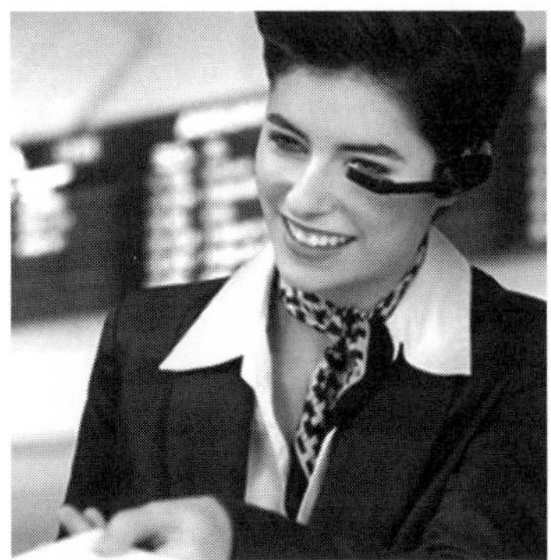

Figure 7-12 Smart-Glasses (M100 Smart Glasses)
Source: Mikimoto, http://www.mikimoto-japan.com/beans/products/m100/index.htm.

in his "office" while talking with "old colleagues."

2.8 Robots that work in collaboration with internet TV programs

A recreation system which consists of various video contents, internet TV programs and a robot "*Sota*" by Vstone was developed by the laboratory of Noriaki Kuwahara at Kyoto Institute of Technology. Then, this system was assessed for its practical value in elderly facilities (Doi, Kuwahara, & Morimoto, 2016). The visual contents provided by the system include physical exercises, reminiscence therapies, and many other recreational activities. The robots can be involved in communication with the participants in each recreational activity. The robot seems to be helpful for the persons who have difficulties in concentrating on visual contents for a certain length of time, such as over 15 minutes. The researchers received many positive comments from staff members in care facilities, saying that using the system provides them with room to breathe both physically and mentally during the recreation time (Figure 7-13).

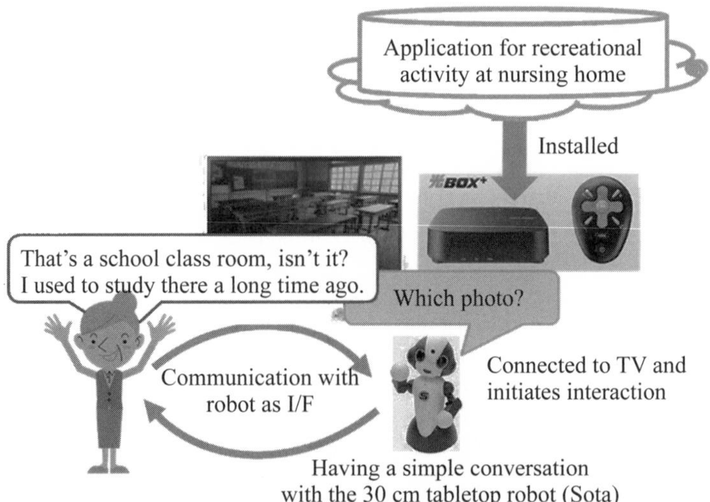

Figure 7-13 Recreation robot working in collaboration with TV monitor

2.9 A mobile agent robot for assisting persons with dementia

The robot "*ilbo*" by Extrun can monitor indoor circumstances, and remote operators make it move in the room as they wish. In some restaurants and hospitals, robots are automatically carrying medicine and food while avoiding pedestrians and tables. On September 2021, Amazon introduced a household robot "Astro" which is squat with two wheels and a rectangular screen. Astro is a big "camera" on wheels that will watch everything that the user does. This kind of robot will become practical in the near future as a moving robot that watches over elderly people.

Meanwhile, the laboratory of Mutsuo Sano at Osaka Institute of Technology, where I work, is developing a mobile agent robot in which an agent on a PC monitor is fixed on a mobile cabinet. The robot is designed to follow a person while providing various assistance in his/her home. Following the person all the time, the robot can observe and record their behavior by attached devices. The role of the robot is to perform like a secretary who always follows and helps the person with dementia.

With this robot, we are planning to provide persons with the following assistance: to give information about the locations where they put their belongings, to mediate videophone conversations between themselves and their remote family members/friends through the PC monitor on the cabinet, and to give timely instructions for them to accomplish daily routines. The robot will be also equipped with drawers for storing belongings, files, and paper documents in order to be easily found later on. Deep learning by AI will allow the robot to recognize automatically what the users have in their hands and what kinds of behavior they perform, to make a summary of recorded conversations with the family members or visitors, and to reply to questions from users based on the summary.

We have succeeded in developing a robot that follows a person by recognizing the skeleton image of the person's back (Riyan, Tanimoto, Sano et al., 2017) (Figure 7-14). Compared with human shaped robots, the robot uti-

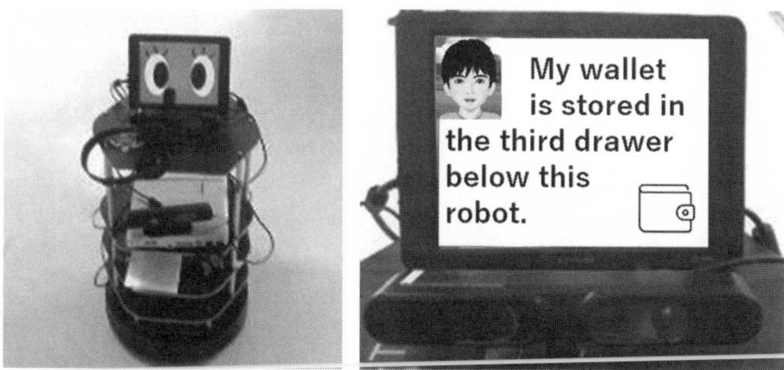

Figure 7-14 Mobile agent robot for assisting persons with dementia

lizing a cabinet is inexpensive, easily modified, and convenient for carrying and managing various belongings and documents in drawers on the cabinet (see Koutentakis, Pilozzi, & Huang (2020) for other information).

2.10 A balloon airship following people and observing their face

Recently, in some elderly facilities, cameras are fixed on the walls or ceilings so that they can detect abnormal postures of the people there and inform staff members of the situation. However, peoples' facial expressions are difficult to follow if they move constantly. If it becomes possible to observe their expressions in real time, it would enable staff members to respond quickly when necessary for the peoples' mental or emotional changes. Srisamosorn, Kuwahara, Yamashita et al. (2016) at the laboratory of Jun Ota at Tokyo University tried to develop a system to observe the facial expressions of people by following them automatically from the air.

The observation was possible by installing a camera onto a balloon airship and following a specified person or a group of people about whom staff members were worried. To be effective, the three-dimensional position of the balloon in the air needs to be determined by synchronizing it with a fish-eye camera on the ceiling. Compared to a drone, a balloon airship can easily be fixed to the ceiling, requires less battery power, and makes almost no noise. It is also possible for persons to feel more accepting of balloon airships than mechanical devices. Another benefit is that a balloon airship can move effortlessly in a home environment whereas robots have difficulty moving over steps, tiny paths, and the stairs between upper and lower floors (Figure 7-15). We expect that this balloon will assist people by providing information from the air.

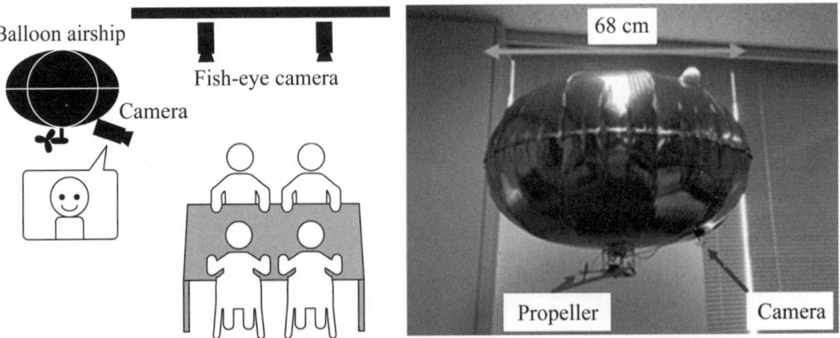

Figure 7-15 Balloon airship following people and observing facial expressions

AEVENA disclosed an idea for an autonomous indoor flying robot "*Aire*" in 2017 (https://fabcross.jp/news/2017/dmln53000004y10b.html). This robot was expected to fly avoiding obstacles, to be controlled by a smartphone or voice commands, to take photos within 360 degrees, and to return to its charger by itself. It will be possible to use it for watching over persons, recording their daily behaviors, and being a conversation partner (Figure 7-16). Amazon announced that during 2021 a drone "Ring Always Home Cam" will be on the market. It is an autonomous flying device which can shoot a video while flying in a house. Persons with MCI or dementia often lack self-awareness of their memory deficits, and thus it would be useful if the robot has functions such as automatic following, recording, searching, and summarizing conversations for those persons (see Astell et al. (2019) and Jotterand et al. (2019) for other information).

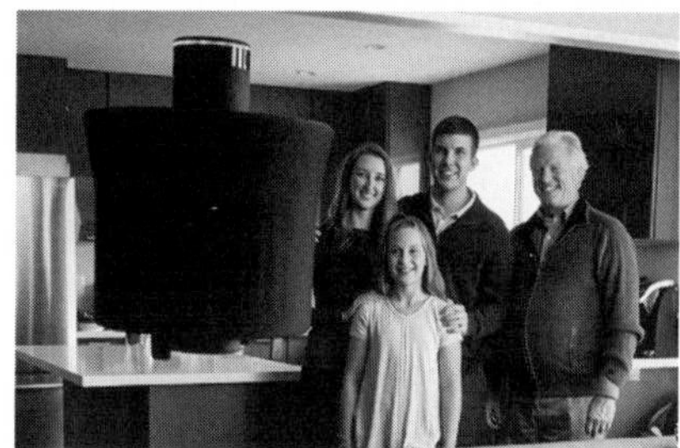

Figure 7-16 Autonomous flying robot "Aire" for indoors
Source: Robotstart, https://robotstart.info/2017/09/26/aevena-aire.html.

3. Dementia-assistance dogs carrying AT devices

As explained so far, High-Tech AT will be able to assist persons with MCI or dementia with tasks which Low and Middle-Tech AT cannot. Some barriers to High-Tech AT use in daily life include the fact that they are expensive, complicated, and require constant maintenance. Hence, family members always need to ask for technical service help when they have trouble with their AT. Furthermore, we face the challenging issues, again, that persons with dementia may forget or refuse to carry the AT, and are not motivated to accept the instructions emitted by the AT. As an innovative solution for these problems, we came up with the idea of employing dogs in collaboration with AT (Yasuda, Kuwahara, Nakamura et al., 2012).

Traditionally, dogs are owned by people as pets. They have also been working for people in various fields. Some jobs require physical strength, mental endurance, heightened attention, and kindness of heart; those are, for example, sled-pulling dogs, guide dogs, hearing dogs, and animal therapy dogs. Recently, there are some studies of training dogs to assist persons with dementia although AT are not used (refer to the website "Dog 4 Dementia"). Our idea is to make dogs follow, look for, and motivate owners or persons with dementia by carrying the AT on their body or collaborating with the AT (Yasuda et al., 2012). With the AT, dogs can provide persons with various types of help with music, videos, and verbal instructions. If the dogs are too small, the AT should be placed on the table or wall, as described later.

If the dog-AT collaboration can be realized, dogs' obedient mind, acute sense of smell and hearing, mobility, and memory ability may become very helpful. The collaboration will make it possible to provide various kinds of assistance for persons with dementia that have been difficult to provide by AT alone. There have been no previous reports of creating the dog-AT collaboration to assist persons with dementia. Fortunately, many owners these days are dressing their dogs in clothing with pockets that can be convenient for carrying medicines or carrying ATs (Figure 7-17).

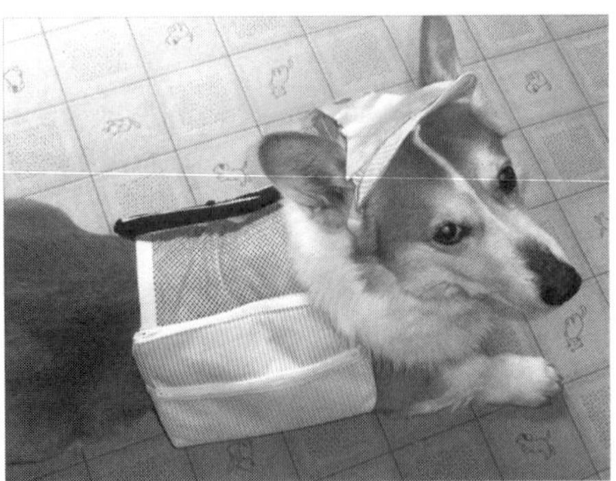

Figure 7-17 Model of dementia-assistance dog carrying AT

Table 7-2 shows examples of the collaboration of dogs and AT. The AT carried by the dogs include devices and items that vary depending on the level of dementia, the ability of the dog, the situation of the owner, and the type of assistance. The dog may carry, for example, a diary, the IC Rec, a smartphone, a camera, or medicines and a bottle of water. The dog will actively behave in collaboration with the AT as follows: hearing sounds out-

Table 7-2 Examples of advantages of collaboration of dogs and AT

Dogs	AT
To look for the owner	To motivate the owner to perform daily routines
To give comfort to the owner	To play favorite videos or music
To follow the owner's behaviors	To record actions in order to locate objects later
To lead the owner	To locate the toilet
To judge whether things/people are known or unknown to the owner	To take photos of the owner and send them to the family after detecting the sound of barking

put automatically from the devices, the dog goes to the owner with items that are already in the pocket of the clothes. If the dog is further trained by its owner, the dog might react to the owner's voice saying the name of the lost belonging and looking for it. The dog follows the owner while recording his/her speech or behaviors by an IC Rec or a camera. The recordings are later played back to find, for example, where the owner placed his/her belongings or what he/she said or was told by family members and visitors. See Yasuda et al. (2012) or our website "The community to train assistance dogs carrying ICT for dementia" (http://hojoken.grupo.jp/) for more detailed information (in Japanese).

At the laboratory of Koichi Nakayama at Saga University, the following experiments were conducted based on two questions (Oshima, Yasuda, Uno et al., 2015): Can a dog learn to go to its owner in response to an auditory alarm? How is the owner's behavior altered by the arrival of the dog? Initially, we trained a dog (a female toy-poodle, five years old) to carry a smartphone on its back. In the first phase, the dog was trained to go to the owner when the smartphone alarm sounded. Every time the dog succeeded in going to the owner, the dog was rewarded with food. It took only three days for the dog to learn this response to the alarm.

In the next phase, we compared the owner's reaction to the smartphone being delivered to him by the dog and when the smartphone was placed in the living room. Previously, we experienced that the messages of IC Rec or smartphone alarms put in the living room were often unnoticed by the elderly; this obviously reduces the effectiveness of the sound-emitting interventions. In the current experiment, therefore, we placed the smartphone on the desk in the living room and asked the dog's owner to turn it off when he/she heard the alarm of the smartphone. The results showed that the owner failed to turn off the alarm 8 out of 17 times. The owner apparently did not notice the alarm while cooking in the kitchen.

Then, as the next step, we had the dog carry the smartphone again on its back. When the sound was emitted, the dog rushed to the owner. The number of failures to turn off the alarm by the owner was reduced to 4 out of 17 times, suggesting that the ratio for achieving daily routines increases when the dog comes to the owner to inform her/him of the routine (Figure 7-18).

A 75-year-old man did not keep a diary in spite of his daughter's repeated instructions for the last several years. An experiment was conducted with his dog (a miniature dachshund, five years old) wearing the IC Rec. It took three days to have the dog learn to respond to the alarm. In order for the owner to fill in his diary, an alarm was automatically emitted from an IC Rec at set times daily. The dog rushed to the owner immediately after hearing it. One minute later, the IC Rec emitted automatically the recorded instruction of his daughter, "Dad, please write in the diary." Although five years have passed since the intervention began, the owner still continues keeping a diary. The owner reported that he felt motivated when the dog came and "asked" him to do a task since he loved dogs.

We tried the same intervention with another dog (a corgi, eight years old) and it took several days to learn to respond to the alarm. We then succeeded in training the dog to bring a "medicine bag" to its owner when the dog heard the alarm. Videos of dogs responding to the alarms are available on my website (https://gensoshi.jimdofree.com/home-pages-for-english/).

Even for advanced robots, it is still difficult for them to follow a person who moves around the house. It would require complicated programs to be

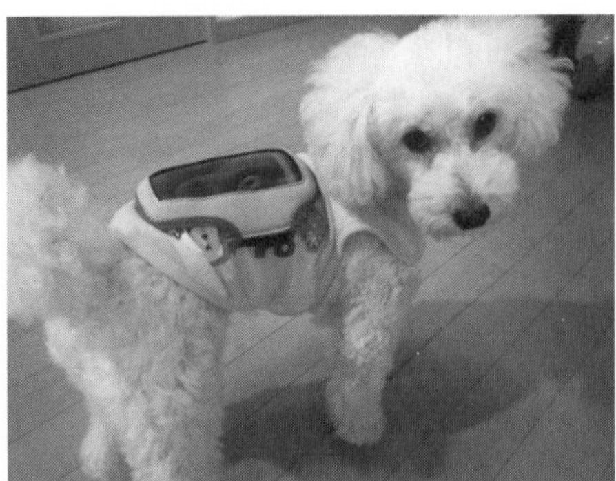

Figure 7-18 Dementia-assistance dog carrying smartphone

written for such a task. However, it may be easier for dogs to locate the person. Dogs can move swiftly, for instance, to upper floors, the garden, even the hills nearby which robots would have difficulty to do. The owner only needs to train the dog with food to reward it for responding to the alarm. If remote family members activate the "videophone" function of a smartphone and sound the alarm (by utilizing **the automatic response function at incoming calls**, see Section 3.3 in Chapter 6), the dog may immediately go and look for the owner. Then, it may become possible for the family members to watch over other members with dementia and have videophone conversations.

The most important advantage in using dogs is that the owners feel much deeper affection for the dogs than other devices such as dolls and robots. Even if the dog cannot work as an assistance dog, caring for dogs and walking with them are soothing and healthy routines for persons with dementia. Many elderly people hesitate to keep dogs because they are worried that they will not be able to take care of them when they have severe dementia or physical impairments. In such cases, neighbors who love dogs or volunteers may take care of their dogs.

Additionally, we conducted a preliminary trial in which a dog tried to "talk" with participants in an elderly facility. The verbal messages were delivered to them from the smartphone on the dog's back. The messages were operated by one of the research members hiding 20 meters away. From the viewpoint of participants, however, it looked as if the dog was speaking (Oshima, Yasuda, Uno et al., 2015). When the dog approached the partici-

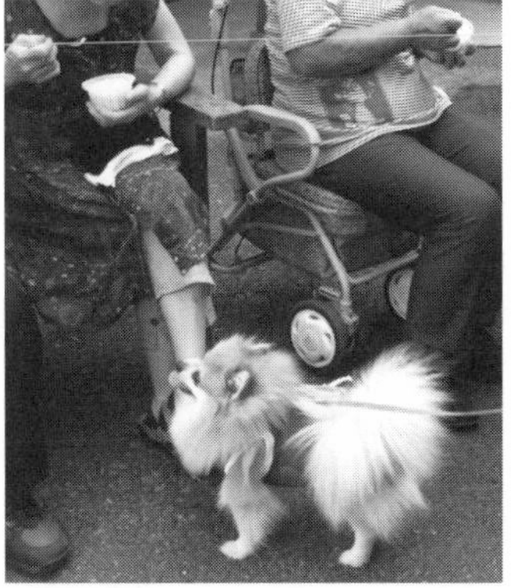

Figure 7-19 Conversation via smartphone on the back of a dementia-assistance dog

pants, they were eating ice cream. The dog said, "I want to eat ice cream with you." The participants looked a little surprised at the beginning, but soon got used to it and said to the dog, "Have you become able to speak the language? Would you like to eat one together?" They seemed to enjoy conversation with the dog (Figure 7-19).

I heard many dog lovers say, "we want to talk with our dogs." Currently, we are planning to carry out experiments to find out whether persons with dementia can enjoy reminiscence conversations with "dogs." If smartphones are installed with the *mago* [grandchild] *anime* agent system (see Section 2.1 in this chapter) and reminiscence questions are emitted from the smartphone on the dog's back, reminiscence conversation might be possible, which may be particularly effective for dog-loving persons.

What is important for this project is to accumulate experiences in trials with combinations of dogs and ATs. A veterinarian said, "Dogs have a habit of following the boss. At the first stage, commands for the dogs would be better to be emitted by a director of the facility." Veterinarians and dog trainers could be involved in this project. We would like to present the results of the trials on our website and get ideas for further improvement. See our homepage and watch demonstration videos of dogs (http://hojoken.grupo.jp/).

In January 2018, SONY launched a dog-shaped robot "*Aibo*" that was designed to read people's facial expressions. Such robots are recommended for elderly dog-lovers to "take care of." In the near future, we will have dog robots that follow owners and read their minds from facial expressions. Then, dog robots will also assist elderly people in various ways as we described earlier in the studies of real dogs and ATs. In some studies, researchers have begun to discover that real dogs elicit different reactions from users when compared to interactions with dog robots. The advantages of real dogs with ATs (or, without ATs), and dog robots should be determined for assisting persons with dementia in their daily lives.

This book described various examples of interventions for assisting persons with MCI and dementia. In fact, there remain many problems of persons for which we still cannot find ways to support them, such as better ways to communicate with persons in no-AT situations, reliable ATs that support safe and comfortable living throughout the day, and ways for persons with dementia to demonstrate loving behaviors towards others. We hope that dementia-assistance dogs will be one of the solutions. We also expect the research of this field will develop into an academic domain called "Human-Computer-Animal-Interface (HCAI)" (Yasuda et al., 2012).

CHAPTER EIGHT

The operation manual for the Memory Clinic, public/regional support, and self/mutual-support

Increasing numbers of persons with dementia live alone without any social support, live taking care of another person with dementia, or live with an unmarried and jobless child. In the anticipation of these situations occurring, the U.K. government in 2005 declared the implementation of a remote support policy for the elderly. I submitted "the Model Project for proactive-measures for dementia" to the Chiba Prefectural office in 2007 as a report of a "workshop on measures for dementia in Chiba Prefecture" (Figure 8-1). In this model project, the following measures were proposed: to subsidize tele-communication costs for the elderly, to support home dwelling persons with dementia through videophones, and to implement lending services of assistive devices for memory impairments.

Eight years later, the Japanese government publicized the policy "the New Orange Plan in 2015," in which the development and implementation of robots and ICTs were proclaimed to be the main plan for caring for persons with dementia. Regrettably, I had to criticize this proclamation in the following four points: first, the extent of effectiveness in using robots is still uncertain for caring for persons with dementia, although it should continue to be studied. Second, prior to the use of robots and ICT, the proliferation of Low-Tech AT which are simple, inexpensive and effective for the persons with dementia should be promoted. Third, videophones that are the most promising supportive ICT were not included in the implementation plan. Fourth, utilizing ICTs or Middle-Tech ATs should be performed in parallel with lending/maintenance services and educational training for ITC literacy. Without exploring these basic technologies and back-up systems, the successful development of practical robots and utilization of ICT to support

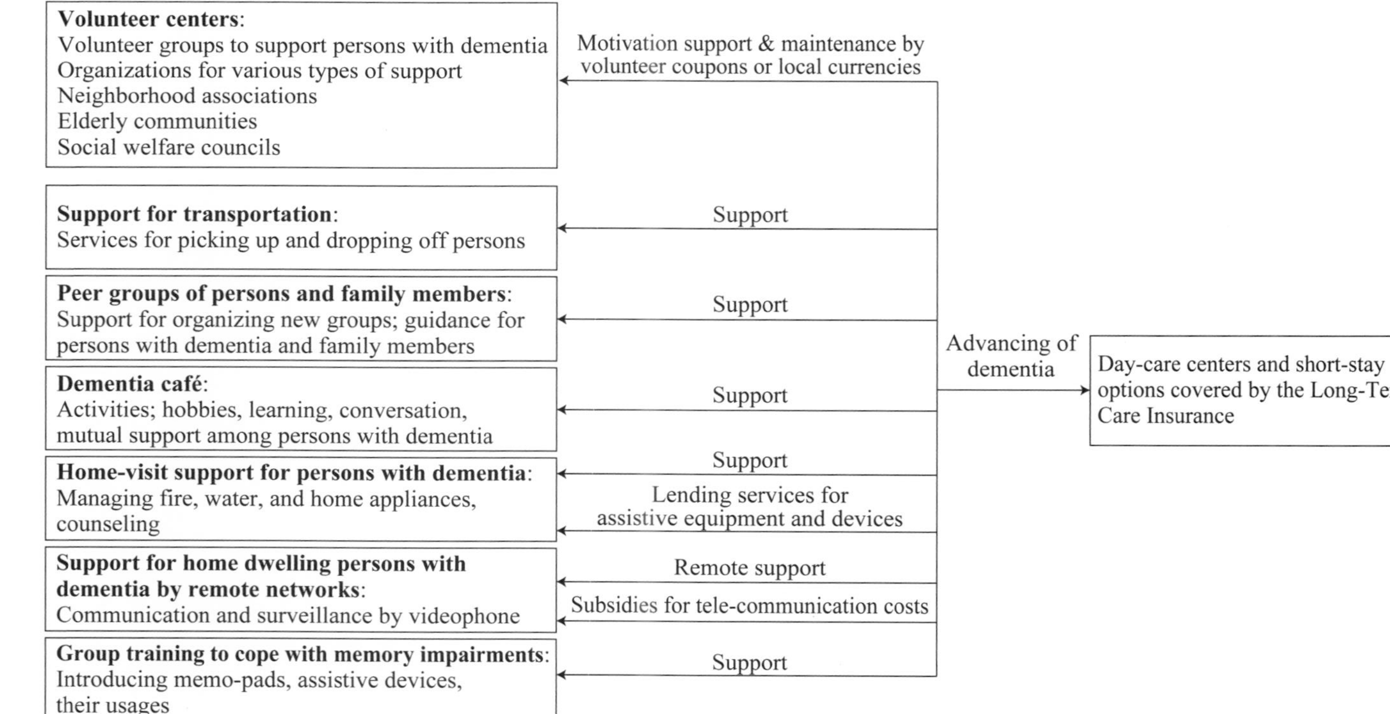

Figure 8-1 Model of proactive-measures for dementia

the daily-life of persons with dementia would be difficult to achieve.

The necessity and effectiveness of remote communication has been proven since the Covid-19 turmoil in 2020. Recently the Japanese government has started reducing tele-communication costs for all generations and providing subsidies for videophone systems at elderly facilities for family members to talk with residents. However, the measures such as providing subsidies for videophones for home dwelling persons and lending services for ATs have not yet begun (see Figure 8-1).

To maintain the daily lives of persons with MCI and dementia, public, regional, and self/mutual support services are important, in addition to an early diagnosis, medications, and rehabilitation. Furthermore, as a form of post-diagnostic support, the Japanese Society of Neurology (2017) recommended the following activities: education about dementia, preparation of a living will, and care plans for persons when independent living becomes difficult.

Narumoto and others are promoting the Collaboration Center of Law, Technology and Medicine for autonomy of older adults (COLTEM) project, which aims to support the decision-making and property management of persons with dementia (Narumoto, 2016; 2017). In order to fulfill this purpose, collaboration is needed among multiple fields, not only medicine, rehabilitation, engineering, public/reginal organizations, and welfare companies, but also finance, insurance, and other private companies. As shown with this project, the range of professionals who participate in dementia support is expanding (see Jotterand et al. (2019) and Sixsmith (2020) for related information).

In order to realize the above support and activities, early detection of MCI and dementia is the first priority. Recently, the number of memory clinics that support early detection of diseases is increasing. Many clinics, however, focus only on testing to detect MCI or dementia and do not recommend rehabilitation approaches or provide information of other possible support services. It may be that detailed operations manuals for rehabilitation approaches have not been published in Japan. This chapter will describe the operations manual of a memory clinic and various types of post-diagnostic support services.

1. The operations manual for the Memory Clinic

This section will describe the operations manual and the manual of rehabilitation approaches utilizing AT for MCI/dementia of the Memory Clinic at the Rehabilitation Department of Chiba Rosai Hospital. As the manual was first compiled at the end of 2017 (Table 8-1), the present manual is different from the manual described below. Therefore, contact me at the address shown at the end of this book if you have any questions about the manual (see Hickey & Bourgeois (2018) for family and professional caregiver's support).

2. Regional support after diagnosis

Even if people are not diagnosed as having MCI or dementia, it is unavoidable that they will suffer deteriorating memory abilities caused by aging. Accordingly, they are given "*Summarized list of memory strategies for the healthy elderly*" as shown in Appendix 4, and "*Detailed list of memory strategies for the healthy elderly*" as in Appendix 5. These resources will help them to prepare for possible troubles caused by declining memory functions as they get older.

Persons diagnosed as having MCI or dementia are also given the above two documents (Appendices 4 and 5). Furthermore, it is explained to them that there are many organizations from which to seek advice, and that they can use various AT, the Long-Term Care Insurance, and other public support services. In addition, there are many regional support groups such as dementia cafés and peer groups of persons and family members. By participating in these activities, they might maintain their activities of daily living and reduce memory problems. The social resources introduced below are examples of the regional support groups and activities in Ichihara City, which my colleagues and I are involved in managing. The item 8 is a model project that promotes disseminating ATs and supports the continuous use of them.

1. "*Oboeteru kai* [the meeting of "do you remember?"]" is a peer group meeting for persons with MCI and mild dementia. Persons and their family members have been getting together once a month since 2007. Around 30 people participate every time. They are divided into groups; each one consisting of about six members. The family members form their own groups. Each group discusses how to deal with problems they have in daily lives. Once a year, they bring their "Ending Notes" to the meeting and try completing "the living will" in their Notes as one of the preparation activities for the end of life. Recently, as the stages of

Table 8-1 Operations manual of the Memory Clinic of Chiba Rosai Hospital

First visit: A reservation is required to visit the Memory Clinic. When clients visit for the first time, they are to complete a medical intake sheet and a questionnaire for forgetfulness (Speedy questionnaire for forgetfulness). The client's family members may complete these forms. Next, an interview by a physician, blood tests, and cognitive assessments by a speech pathologist are performed. An MRI brain image may be taken on another day; the degree of atrophy of the parahippocampal gyrus and cerebrum are measured by the VSRAD (Voxel-based Specific Regional analysis system for Alzheimer's Disease; Matsuda, 2007)
Cognitive assessment battery: A Speech Language Pathologist (SLP) conducts the cognitive assessment battery as described in Chapter 1. If the family members observe the client taking the tests, they may learn about his/her current cognitive abilities by how he/she responds to the questions. If the client is suspected to have depression or dementia with Lewy bodies, the GHQ test or the Noise pareidolia test are added, respectively. The results are summarized on "Results of the cognitive assessment battery." and will be reviewed at the Diagnostic Summary Conference.
Diagnostic Summary Conference: Professionals such as doctors of related departments, SLPs, nurses, and counselors gather at a conference held once a week to discuss the clinical conditions of each client who visited the Memory Clinic. Diagnoses are decided based on the results of tests and other materials mentioned above. The following factors are also discussed: whether the client has depression, side effects from medications, and other co-morbidities. If he/she has MCI or dementia, the type, severity, potential medicines and rehabilitation approaches, and short term outcomes are discussed. The team may recommend additional tests such as SPECT (Single Photon Emission Computed Tomography) and MIBG (Meta-iodobenzylguanidine) in order to differentiate symptoms of MCI from normal aging and Lewy bodies dementia. If consensus about a definite diagnosis cannot be reached, the diagnosis is put on hold. The client is asked to come to the Memory Clinic again in six months or one year to retake the assessment battery.
Interviews by SLPs: Some clients are aware of their forgetfulness in daily life, but many persons with dementia say, "I came here because my family members think I have memory problems." We ask family members and the client, if possible, to complete the speedy questionnaire for forgetfulness. By examining the responses, differences in their responses become apparent. The fact that some family members cannot appropriately evaluate the client's memory and cognitive abilities when they are living separately, has to be considered in making a diagnosis. Family members should be interviewed in separate rooms in order to reveal their real intentions. During the interview with the family members, the client has a conversation with a volunteer companion.

Points of observation:
The SLP should monitor whether the client repeats the same stories during the examinations since this reflects the severity of forgetfulness. Pay attention to how they walk when they enter and leave the room because an abnormal gait may indicate the possibility of having vascular dementia or Lewy body dementia. Observe the expression of their face. Clients without facial affect may have fewer social interaction opportunities in their daily lives. Also observe the facial expressions of the family members and their behaviors to infer their relationship with the client. It may be possible to assume the attitudes of family members towards what neighbors and acquaintances say about the client. These attitudes may be related to their acceptance of regional supports.

Reporting of diagnoses:
The doctor explains to the client and the family members the diagnosis discussed in the Diagnostic Summary Conference, the pathology of the disease, an outline of treatment, and prescription of medicines. Then, the SLP explains to the persons being diagnosed with MCI/dementia and family members about the following matters in detail: the results of the cognitive assessment battery, instructions for coping with memory impairments, description of AT and lending services, plans for periodic testing, the application for "*kaigo hoken*" (the Long-Term Care Insurance), and the many public institutions for social support services.

In addition, the SLP will inform them of peer groups of persons with dementia/family members, counselling by telephone, hobby groups, and other regional resources as described later. The SLP encourages them to make the most of the above resources and to accept various supports without hesitation. Finally, the SLP tells them that the goal of rehabilitative approaches is to maintain or to recover QOL of the person/family members by incorporating various supports and utilizing AT. It may take approximately one and a half hour for the SLP to report and explain the above results. A copy of "the results of the cognitive assessment battery" will be given to them if they wish. The SLP may tape-record the explanations of the results for other family members who were unable to attend on that day.

Persons with MCI and mild dementia are given the following documents (see Appendices): "*Consent Form on Surveillance for MCI/dementia and Helping Each Other*," "*Dementia Declaration and Request Form for Assistance*," "*Summarized List of Memory Strategies for the Healthy Elderly*," "*Detailed List of Memory Strategies for the Healthy Elderly*" (described later). We also give them booklets about general information on dementia provided by pharmaceutical companies.

The cognitive assessment battery will be administered again in a few months, six months, or one year, depending on their condition. If the scores of the retest are found to have deteriorated, doctors will review the severity of dementia, the prescribed amount and types of medicines, as well as the addition of new medicines. The test scores of some persons may not show any change for several years, while some may worsen consistently over time or suddenly. Unpredictable changes in the symptoms of MCI/dementia may require periodic examination as well as inquiring about their ADL and QOL.

In order to advise about activities of daily living, SPLs may ask the following questions to confirm the situations, and discuss with them how to improve or maintain their daily lives:

1. Who takes care of the person's medicine?
2. Do you use an IH system in the kitchen? In case a gas oven is used, are dry-heating protection sensors installed?
3. Are fire alarm sensors equipped?
4. Does the water supply to the bathtub stop automatically?
5. Who takes care of the person's banking?
6. Is an "answering machine" for the phone activated?
7. Do the person and family members use smartphones, tablets, and/or PCs? Are they connected to the Internet? Is a GPS tracking function installed on the smartphones?
8. Who does the shopping? Or, are delivery services used?
9. Has the person fallen to the floor/ground? Is the person getting sufficient physical exercise including walking?
10. What are other difficult problems for which they would like to get advice?

Assistive Technologies (AT):

SLPs introduce the redirection techniques and compensatory AT approaches to cope with various memory-related problems in their daily activities. The following AT are available in the Memory Clinic: Sony IC Recorders (ICD-PX240), locating and tracking devices for lost objects, electronic/non-electronic medicine boxes, timers, human detection sensors and voice-emitting devices, tablets, blackboards, surveillance cameras, DVD players, DVDs for reminiscence therapy, digital photo frames, sound amplifiers for hearing difficulties, dolls, memo-pads, calendars and message boards, pedometers, and other Low Tech-AT (introduced in Chapters 2 and 5). The SLP introduces some AT which may fit the needs of the person and family members according to the clinical stage.

In many cases, they have no experience of using the above AT. Thus, the devices are often loaned to the person after setting up the system. They are advised to purchase some AT later on when they find using them useful.

Others:

The instructions for how to use the AT should be written down and given to persons and family members. The written notes are necessary because it is difficult for most of them to learn the instructions and other information at one time. Furthermore, after being told the diagnosis they might become too distressed to remember anything.

At the next visit, the SPL asks them what problems still remain to be resolved after trying the previous recommendations. Further instructions may be given to them, or other ways of coping may be discussed with them. If AT was loaned to them, the SLP asks how they have been using the devices. If the effectiveness of the AT was not as good as expected, the SLP may reconsider the usage of them or recommend other AT. This trial and error guidance will be conducted whenever they come to the Memory Clinic. Then, a written memo of the schedule for the next appointment is given to the person. A clerk of the clinic usually gives a reminder call to the person who lives alone prior to the clinic visit.

MCI or dementia of the participants have been progressing, the discussion about particular topics is becoming difficult. Archives of the last 15 years are found on the blog of this group (https://blogs.yahoo.co.jp/monowasurekondankai). This blog contains "*Oboeteru kai News*" which record difficulties experienced by persons with MCI or dementia and by their family members, and advice for coping methods. The records will be valuable resources for researchers in developing novel AT.

2. Consultation Café for forgetfulness/dementia is held once a month. The purpose of the Café is mainly for personal consultations to discuss problems caused by MCI and dementia. Participants may talk with an SLP, nurse, and/or care manager while having coffee. There are also lectures on using AT; the contents of the lectures differ every month.
3. Consultation Café for PC/smartphones opens at the same time and place as the above 2, where a volunteer specialist holds consultations for visitors who have problems with ICT devices and applications of smartphones. If they bring their device to the Café the specialist can evaluate and fix any problem they are having with the device. Launching this kind of counseling and support service for ICT is definitely required for promoting AT or ICT for persons with MCI/dementia, family members, as well as for the healthy elderly. Therefore, normally aging citizens are welcomed to the Café.
4. Consultation "Pub" for persons with dementia and family members is a meeting to discuss coping with various problems while drinking and eating at a *sushi* bar once every two months. Remote consultation is simultaneously held by Skype or Zoom for the participants who cannot come to the site due to living far away or being unable to leave a person with dementia alone at home.
5. An online chat-room for persons with MCI/other diseases is held every Wednesday at 5:00 pm. Further, an online chat-room for family members is also open every second Tuesday at 2:30 pm, once every two months. Currently, there are about five and seven participants, respectively.
6. A training course for "*Monowasure* [Memory] *Supporters*" is the system we developed for promoting AT literacy in 2019. The training courses are for professionals in the care, medical, and welfare fields and citizens who are interested in utilizing AT for persons with MCI/dementia or for themselves. The Memory Supporter is a newly created certification aiming at proliferating the knowledge of AT to professionals in related fields and citizens.

The designation of Memory Supporter is classified into three grades. The 3rd-grade Memory Supporters are to share the knowledge of AT learned in the course with their peers in smaller meetings. The 2nd-grade Memory Supporters are expected to hold training courses using predetermined teaching materials and to provide support activities for persons with MCI or dementia. The 1st-grade Memory Supporters are eligible to foster and supervise 2nd- and 3rd-grade Memory Supporters. The training course is usually composed of six day programs where participants learn how to deal with persons with forgetfulness and MCI/dementia by using AT. When they complete the course, they are qualified to take an exam for the certification of Memory Supporter. If they pass the exam, they will be certified as Memory Supporter (3rd-grade). There are about six 2nd- and fifty 3rd-grade Memory Supporters as of 2021.

They are required to take an exam every four years to learn new AT and renew the certification. We currently plan to hold remote courses for training Memory Supporters. Please check the HP for more information (https://memorysupporter.jimdofree.com/).

7. The Liaison Council for Countermeasures against dementia in Ichihara City (http://ichininkyo.grupo.jp/) was established in 2014 by organizing professionals in a wide range of related fields, including medicine, nursing, welfare, peer groups, and city government. The number of members is approximately 200. Currently, it consists of eight project teams to discuss eight countermeasures. As one of the enlightenment projects for citizens, an "*Ichihara dementia fair*" has been held annually since 2017 with a total of 20 booths and many small lectures. More than 250 citizens come to the fair. The liaison council also introduces other social resources in the city on its HP to the public.
8. The peer group of family members for dementia in our city (*Hanamizuki no kai*) holds a monthly meeting, where approximately 30 people participate including professional caregivers, care managers, volunteers, and others. Sometimes they invite lecturers to speak on relevant topics.
9. I proposed a model project that promotes disseminating AT and supports the continuous use of them. It was submitted to Ichihara City in September 2020 as one of the policies for "After Covid 19." Even after the pandemic of Covid 19, the shortage of professional caregivers will remain. The number of elderly, as well as persons with dementia, will definitely increase. Utilization of AT for them should be backed up by close cooperation between related professionals in the city (Figure 8-2).

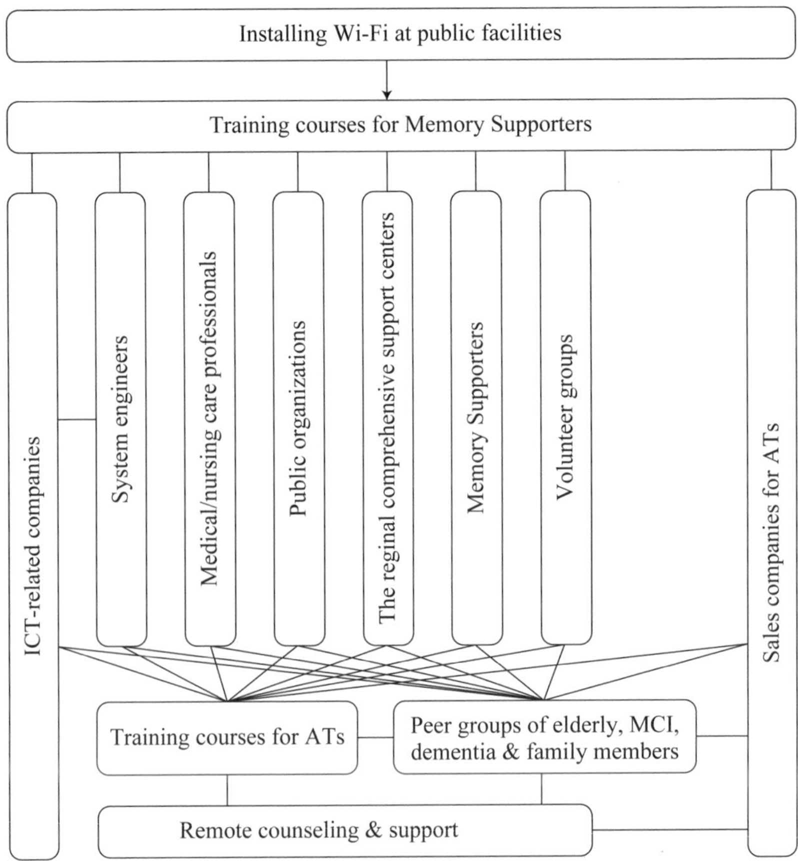

Figure 8-2 Model project for dissemination of AT
Note: AT = Assistive Technologies.

3. Self- and mutual-support services

The Long-Term Care Insurance of Japan aims to support the activities of daily living (ADL)of home dwelling persons with dementia and family members. The government states that more services should be supplied for home care. The current policy, however, is discouraging people from using the insurance by tightening the applicable conditions. The government seems to abandon its responsibility as the main "public" supporter. Instead, it is asking for self- and mutual-support among the elderly people with the help of volunteers, local associations, NPOs, and others. We should continue criticizing the government's policy.

Meanwhile, the Japanese Society of Neurology (2017) stated that the following written declarations are necessary, although further and deliberate discussion is needed: (1) the living will expressing your end of life wishes (see Hickey & Bourgeois (2018) for more information on end of life issues), and (2) the support you want to receive if diagnosed as having dementia. I have compiled the above related documents (drafts) for a living will, dementia declarations, and self- and mutual-support. You may use them by altering them as you like since you need to consider the differences in culture and circumstances of persons, families, friends, and place of residence. The following documents can be printed out from my website (search with "Kiyoshi Yasuda homepage").

3.1 Forms for detecting MCI/dementia in various situations (draft) (Appendix 1)

Many forms or checking list for detecting MCI/dementia are available today. The series of forms I created (Appendix 1), however, differ from traditional forms and can be used in various daily situations. The series contains eight different forms according to the situations such as at shops, at banks, at pharmacies, at dentists/hospitals, at barbers/hairdressers, at social circles, at delivery services, and in neighborhoods. These forms will help relevant members in each field to detect the early-onset of MCI or dementia of customers, friends, and neighbors. The evaluation items of each form were prepared with the advice of members in the field.

When a member involved in each field notices abnormal forgetfulness of someone the results of the form can be communicated to the person, a family member, or the regional comprehensive support center. These forms may be useful in particular for persons who live alone and lack self-awareness of their forgetfulness. Appendix 2 is an example of the "barbers/ hairdressers" form. These forms are available on my website.

3.2 Consent form on mutual surveillance for MCI/dementia and helping each other (draft) (Appendix 2)

When the stage of an individual's forgetfulness progresses, his/her friends may notice increased frequency of forgetfulness. This is a consent form on mutual surveillance for MCI and dementia. You and your friend are to make a promise in advance that when one notices the other's worsening memory, he/she should point it out to the other. A person who is told by a friend may be more likely to see a doctor at a memory clinic. Furthermore, they will help each other after a diagnosis of having MCI or dementia. As many people often refuse to recognize their forgetfulness when it is pointed out by family members, this system involving friends is expected to work better.

There was a newspaper article about 15 ex-co-workers who made up a support team for a woman, their former colleague, with early-onset dementia. They helped her by sharing the opportunities to assist her with her daily routines and events, for example, accompanying her to the hospital (*Asahi Shimbun* [newspaper], February 15, 2017).

If the consent form is signed in advance among friends, a supportive team can be started in advance of an emergency need. Because the amount of public support, such as the Long-Term Care Insurance, is being reduced, it will be wiser to build this kind of mutual assistance system at the earliest convenience while you are still healthy. Once the function of remote operation on your smartphone or PC is installed, a videophone-network, for example, with your family and friends can be easily set up to operate.

3.3 Dementia declaration and request form for assistance (draft) (Appendix 3)

Today, the number of people who disclose having dementia is on the increase. It may be difficult to know if the person you are talking to now has mild dementia and what kind of support is required. This can lead to misunderstandings among friends about missed meetings, returning borrowed money and other sensitive matters. In order to deal with these problems, I created a dementia declaration and a request form for assistance. The form contains a brief explanation of the diseases, troubles persons may have, and of what kind of help they might need. Persons may modify the form as needed when their situation changes. Family members may share the form with people who are willing to help. In the case of MCI, you should change the wording and make an MCI version referring to the dementia form.

3.4 Summarized list of memory strategies for the healthy elderly (Appendix 4)

Even if you do not have dementia, you may not avoid becoming forgetful as you get older. People who already have MCI may experience difficulties in learning to use AT and preparing for the end of life. You need, therefore, to begin, while you are still healthy, to use AT and write a living will of what you hope for the end of your life. What's important is to get accustomed to executing such activities before you have MCI or dementia. This is the summary of Appendix 5. If you are interested in getting more information, see Appendix 5.

3.5 Detailed list of memory strategies for the healthy elderly (Appendix 5)

The activities and coping methods for MCI and dementia discussed at the "*Oboeteru kai*" were edited into a brochure called "I forgot again! A manual for coping with forgetfulness" (2012: available from the website, https://monowasurekondankai.seesaa.net/). It is a booklet of collected ideas to reduce the incidence of forgetfulness by improving daily habits and using Low-Tech and Middle-Tech AT. Ogisawa (2015) also proposed various approaches to prevent forgetfulness. Information in Appendix 5 is a combination of our brochure (2012) and Ogisawa's (2015), as well as a description of additional new AT and goods. We encourage you to use the list at meetings of the healthy elderly, such as exercise classes and hobby classes, to enlighten them about coping methods for forgetfulness.

4. Useful websites and paid services

The most important instruction for persons with dementia and their family members is to seek advice from the relevant organizations before problems occur, since people who try to cope with problems of dementia alone or only with family members often become overwhelmed by the problems as time passes. From our experience, male family members often take longer to accept regional or public supports. Table 8-2 shows useful websites and paid services in Japan. If you find the Long-Term Care Insurance is not enough to support the person, you may use paid services for surveillance or conversation services. Recently, some companies provide a life insurance policy for dementia. To carry such insurance in advance is one of the guarantees to get financial resources for persons with dementia and family members in their later years.

Table 8-2 Useful websites and paid services

Counseling agencies:

- "The regional comprehensive support centers" and "the qualified medical centers for dementia diseases" throughout Japan
- "Dementia care information network" http://www.dcnet.gr.jp/
- "Learning about dementia and living with dementia e-65.net" http://www.e-65.net/
- "Nakamaaru" https://nakamaaru.asahi.com. This is an information site by *Asahi Shimbun* [newspaper] for people living with dementia to continue their own way of life with their family members, friends and communities. In this site, various supportive activities are introduced with many photos and comics.
- A website "*Ninchisho Chienowa* [dementia puzzle ring] *net*" https://chienowa-net.com/. With an aim of reducing the burden on family members, Chienowa net publishes the success probability of coping methods for various symptoms occurring in persons with dementia (Kosugi, Sato, Yoshiyama et al., 2020). Since its launch in 2015, the site has seen a steady increase in the number of registered users and amount of access. Kazui, Sato, Yoshiyama et al. (2020) analyzed 2003 of family members' experiences (male 808, female1192). Appropriate countermeasures that can alleviate responsive behaviors are proposed. The majority of countermeasures are the redirection techniques.
- "Enkyori kaigo [remote care] ranking" https://care.blogmura.com/care_enkyori/ranking/in. It is important to know what services, facilities and surveillance tools are effective for adult children who support their parents remotely. There are many remote family member blogs that talk about various experiences. This site is a ranking site for those blogs.

Societies of persons with dementia, societies of family members:

- "Society of persons with dementia and their families" http://www.alzheimer.or.jp/
- "Society of persons with early-onset dementia: Hoshino kai" http://star2003.mdn.ne.jp/
- "Support network for persons with Lewy body dementia" http://dlbsn.org/
- "Dementia Alliance International (DAI)" https://www.dementiaallianceinternational.org/about-dai/. DAI was established in 2014 to promote education and awareness about dementia. The aim is to eradicate discrimination, improve the QOL of persons with dementia, and urge the government, private sector, and medical professionals to listen to concerns of persons with dementia.

Adult guardianship, living wills, inheritance:

- "Houterasu [legal terrace]" http://www.houterasu.or.jp/. This organization is to provide citizens with information and service guidance they need to solve their legal problems.

Paid services

- "Duskin lifecare" https://lifecare.duskin.jp/
- "Nichii life" http://www.nichiiweb.jp/kaji/
- "Care at home Yasashii-te" http://www.yasashiite.com/index.html

Other surveillance services are performed by the post office, convenience store chains, home-delivery companies.

4.1 Summary

Staff members in memory clinics should inform persons with MCI/dementia and their family members about the availability of various kinds of AT and public/regional supports as post-diagnostic interventions. Smiles often return to their faces after receiving this guidance. Some of them may become positive in thinking about their disease realizing that there are many means to get support that they can rely on hereafter. Therefore, clinical experts should make an effort to improve public/regional resources, not limited to medical support.

On the first day of the "*Oboeteru kai*" (Section 2 in this chapter) in 2007, a male participant asked me with a sad face, "Do I have dementia?" Before I tried to explain it, another participant immediately said to him, "Of course! That's why we gathered here." I worried about his reaction, but to my surprise he responded with a big smile, "Now I understand! I had been wondering about it." This episode tells us the importance of having peers with the same disease.

I have also experienced that not only persons with MCI/dementia, but also the healthy elderly, are confused about what to do about forgetfulness or MCI/dementia, and thus the documents shown in Appendices 1–5 were compiled (although they may need more revisions). We made Appendices 4 and 5 particularly for the healthy elderly, hoping that they are helpful for their preparation for MCI/dementia. It is more important to "prepare for" than to "prevent" MCI and dementia since many people may experience these conditions in their later years. In conclusion, I summarized my thoughts for persons with dementia and their family members as the "Song of Dementia." See next page.

Related Topics —Song of dementia—

I created the following song originally as one of the enlightenment activities in "Workshop on measures for dementia in Chiba Prefecture" in 2007. Please alter the words as you wish to fit a well-known song in your culture and try singing with your peers, persons and family members!

1. No matter how you try to prevent having dementia, it's often useless. Don't hesitate to go to a memory clinic.
2. Now, medicines are prescribed. They won't work if delayed. Take them as soon as the doctor recommends. Then, find your legal guardian.
3. If you hate to go to hospital, make a call for free consultation. Friendly voices of peers and family members wait for you.
4. If you have time to mourn, think of coping methods for forgetfulness. Wearable memo-pads, electronic devices, and smartphones tell you when to take your medicine and the way to go home.
5. Dementia may cause depression while hiding and worrying alone. Instead, day-care centers provide a pick-you-up, bath, lunch, and fun chatting with friends.
6. That's strange. My friend forgets promises very often recently. I will not abandon my friend, as I may also suffer dementia someday.
7. No support can cause abuse and nursing care hell. Do not be afraid, we can help each other. Let's believe in tomorrow's smile.

by Kiyoshi Yasuda, June 16, 2021

Conclusion and advice for the future

The prevention and treatment of dementia, in particular the neurodegenerative types such as Alzheimer's disease or dementia with Lewy bodies, is an ongoing research endeavor. Slowly, scientists are learning more about the underlying causes of, and possible treatments for the disease. But much more evidence is still needed. In the meantime, this book offers practical ways to address the challenging problems of persons with MCI and dementia.

Memory impairment is the core symptom of MCI, dementia, and even normal aging. It is **the information impairment** that can be addressed with Low, Middle, and High-Tech AT (assistive technology). Adopting **the strategy of presenting information in advance** is recommended in order to maintain access to important information for daily living.

Different approaches are suggested for persons at various stages. The healthy elderly are advised to do exercises, adopt healthy living practices to avoid lifestyle-related diseases, and to use strategies to reduce forgetfulness. When early signs of MCI appear, the use of Low-Tech AT may improve their daily functioning. As they experience increasing difficulty with recall of their daily schedule and other information, they can use Middle-Tech AT. And, when their symptoms become more severe, their environments should be adapted in order to enjoy a variety of stimuli such as music, images for reminiscence, videophone conversation, and virtual reality technology. These interventions may help prevent challenging problems at each stage.

Whatever the case, for the following reasons for Low- and Middle-Tech AT, it is recommended that everyone:

- Start using Low-Tech AT now because it is likely that devices that are familiar will continue to be used successfully if you develop MCI or dementia;
- Become familiar with Middle-Tech AT before you need them when your memory function deteriorates;
- Use the automatic features of AT, such as recorded messages from the IC Recorder or the automatic start of the videophone conversation; and
- Use the verbal command feature of some AT or electronic appliances (e.g., smartphones and smart display).

Recently, many elderly people may already have experience with smartphones and some IT devises. Therefore, they will be able to maintain the use of these devices for some time if they develop MCI or dementia in the future.

Professionals should provide AT that are appropriate for each individual's remaining memory, cognitive abilities and circumstances, at each stage. They should also accumulate evidence of the successes and failures of each person's use of AT in order to learn how to develop more suitable AT for future individuals.

Until now, many coping strategies have been proposed on the premise that persons with dementia and family members are living together. However, the number of elderly people living alone, or couples with dementia is increasing. For this reason, this book has introduced many ATs and strategies that can be used by people living alone.

In these days, there are opportunities for remote manipulation of electronic appliances and remote surveillance when help is needed. In Chapter 6, examples of online user groups were described, such as LINE or Facebook. Originally the group's members were supposed to be the user's acquaintances. New groups, however, have been created which aim to help known and unknown persons in their remote local communities. A registered supporter in one of these online groups may offer assistance to any person with dementia who needs help.

A "global network for videophone users with dementia" was also described in Chapter 6. In this network, persons with MCI or mild dementia may assist other persons and serve as conversation companions. Even with the time differences between countries, "conversation at midnight" and "24-hour videophone chat room" are possible. Fortunately, online meeting applications such as ZOOM and Teams have been developed recently. In SpatialChat, participants can create as many groups as they like on a screen, just like a cocktail party.

An example of a support system could be an "AT center," where popular AT are prepared and loaned to users (Astell et al., 2019). AT professionals would be available to recommend AT in consideration of users' desires, abilities, and circumstances. It is important, therefore, to train AT professionals and volunteer assistants who are competent at recommending AT. We have started an experimental training course for "Memory Supporters." They assist by setting up devices and may visit a user's home to provide advice about specific devices and network systems. AT database and special apps should be developed to help these staffs search appropriate ATs for each user. Experts are not always able to yield new ideas of AT. In the above activities, some amateurs may come up with ideas for better AT.

The aim of these programs is to extend the period of time persons with dementia continue to live independently. The frequency of hospitalization and admittance to residential facilities could also be reduced or delayed. The government would be wise to invest more funds to proliferate AT, considering the possible reduction of health/care expenses with a more independent population.

The magazine *AERA* (November, 2015, vol. 47) issued the feature story, "We can work even if we have dementia." The conclusion was that further studies of AT and AT lending services should allow persons with dementia to continue working.

In the future, persons with progressive dementia my benefit from High-Tech AT such as personal agents, "follow-me" home robots, or dementia-assisting dogs carrying ICT devises to assist with their daily activities while utilizing their physiological, behavioral, emotional, and environmental data. Meanwhile, their opinion and preferences should be incorporated. Automatic support systems for excretion, taking a bath, and changing clothes will be realized in the next 20 years.

I overheard a doctor in a memory clinic saying that, "Early detection of dementia means early despair, so the early detection is useless." This argument is not in line with the above viewpoints. Therefore, I would like to suggest changing his words into, "Early detection of dementia enables early usage of AT that will insure continued independence in ADL." In order to detect MCI/dementia, it is necessary to develop assessment methods for the healthy elderly to find subtle deterioration of memory since it may progress to MCI over the years.

Needless to say, AT usage may not solve all of the problems caused by dementia. And, all of the potential effects of AT are still unknown. For example, there are emotional behaviors that may not be modifiable with AT, such as persecution paranoia, hateful feelings towards others, and mood disorders. These behaviors require the prompt and appropriate responses of another human being who can anticipate the persons' needs and provide sympathetic support.

Even if an AT-intervention works well for only one out of 100 persons with dementia, it is a significant success for that person. From a global viewpoint, it means that it is effective for one million out of 100 million persons with dementia. For the remaining 99 or 99 million persons, we should continue seeking other effective methods. I would be very happy if this book provides some reduction in the despair of persons with MCI and dementia, in the burden of their family members, and uncovers clues for improving their independent ADL and QOL.

Dementia has been described as one of the most important issues in the 21st century. We are the innovators to solve these problems, be it slowly but steadily and creatively.

Afterword

My father was a fisherman in Kamogawa City on the coast of the Pacific Ocean. He lost both of his legs in his 40s due to a disease called gangrene. I used to find him looking outside through a crack in the *shoji*-paper screen. The sea was very close to our house, but the road ran in front of the house and the sea was across the street. There was also another house blocking his view of the sea. So, he only heard the sounds of the waves. He was mostly independent in his activities of daily living in spite of his amputations. For example, when he worked in the garden, he moved himself by sliding on his hips. But, it was unsafe for him to move that way to cross the road. If he had had a wheelchair he could have gone to see the sea. My family did not have the money to purchase one, and there were no public services to lend a wheelchair at that time. However, I knew nothing about wheelchairs since I had never seen one.

People may have disabilities of various kinds (i.e., physical, cognitive, etc.) and for many reasons (i.e., preventable or unavoidable). They should be informed that there are compensatory tools (e.g., wheelchairs, prosthetic legs, etc.) and public lending services for persons with disabilities. If such tools or lending services do not exist in a specific location, we should advocate to create them. A fisherman must feel sad if he/she is unable to see the sea. It may be also true for farmers who cannot see their farms. I still feel regret for my father's situation, even after 50 years.

In the movie *The Last Emperor*, there was a scene where Emperor Puyi, who had myopic vision, was advised to wear glasses by his western tutor. His maids, however, opposed this idea strongly, saying, "You should never use such a western tool." At that time, as wheelchairs and eyeglasses were rarely available, family members carried people with walking disabilities on their backs or guided them by holding their hands. There were no other alternatives. Today, it is common for people with such disabilities to use wheelchairs, glasses, and other aids. Consequently, they are now able to live independently. Around 2003, an electronic medicine dispenser was sold on the market. It was an excellent device and it could also be rented at low cost. The media and professionals, however, showed little interest in the product, and its sale was eventually discontinued. We cannot laugh at the maids of Emperor Puyi!

As introduced in this book, the kinds of AT (Assistive Technology) to compensate for the forgetfulness of persons who are aging or have MCI/dementia are increasing. But many people, even professionals in health-related fields, are not familiar with these tools. Accordingly, the AT that are loaned are limited to those for physical impairments. This is the same situation as with wheelchairs 50 years ago. Imagine a life of inconvenience without knowing about the availability of an AT, such as a pair of glasses. Let's ask the government to start a lending service for AT while reducing the cost by utilizing care insurance. Let's ask, also, health professionals to create a section in their journals or publications for introducing AT for MCI/dementia.

In the lecture on February 2017 by Tomofumi Tanno, who had early-onset dementia, he said, "Since I was diagnosed as having dementia, I have been told about my disease and the Long-Term Care Insurance, but no one ever has asked me what I'd like to do from now and what kind of dreams I have." I was one of those professionals who asked the persons with dementia about their "problems" but never asked about their "dreams." So it was painful for me to hear what he was saying.

Meanwhile, his lecture reminded me of a person, whom had a deterioration of memory and muscular strength in his lower limbs. The etiology of the disease was not known at that time, and he and his wife looked distressed. So, I told them, "Unfortunately, it is not helpful to think about what even the newest medical science can't explain. Instead, I'd recommend you take an overseas trip to distract you from your worries?" Soon after, they began visiting World Heritage sites including the Pyramids and Angkor Wat, while the person was in a wheelchair. To my surprise, they went to see the Moai statues on Easter Island. Even with a wheelchair, you can fly to see an island in the middle of the Pacific Ocean!

References

Abe, S. (2017). Saishinno jyouhou gijyutsu wo riyoushita koureisha no seikatsu-shien [Life support for the elderly using the latest information technology]. *Keisoku to Seigyo* [Journal of the Society of Instrument and Control Engineers], 56 (3), 212–215. (In Japanese)

American Psychiatric Association (2013). The diagnostic and statistical manual of mental disorders (5th ed.: DSM-5). https://psycnet.apa.org/record/2013-14907-000.

Anzen unten shien kyokai [Safety driving support association] (2012). *Untenji ninchi shougai souki hakken check list.* [Checklist for early detection of cognitive impairment during driving]. http://sdsd.jp/untenjiniunchisyougai/checklist30/. (in Japanese)

Arai, I. (2006). *Alzheimer no subetega wakaru hon* [A book that tells you everything about Alzheimer's disease]. Kodansha. (In Japanese)

Arai, Y., Kudo, K., Hosokawa, T., Washio, M., Miura, H., & Hisamichi, S. (1987). Reliability and validity of the Japanese version of the Zarit Caregiver Burden Interview. *Psychiatry & Clinical Neuroscience*, 51 (5), 281–287. https://doi.org/10.1111/j.1440-1819.1997.tb03199.x.

Asada, T. (2016). *Senmoni ga oshieru ninchisho* [Dementia explained by a specialist]. Gentosha. (In Japanese)

Baddeley, A. (1995). The psychology of memory. In A. D. Baddeley, B. A. Wilson, & F. N. Watts (Eds.), *Handbook of memory disorders* (pp. 3–26). NY: John Wiley.

Bahar-Fuchs, A., Clare, L., & Woods, B. (2013). Cognitive training and cognitive rehabilitation for mild to moderate Alzheimer's disease and vascular dementia. *Cochrane Database of Systematic Reviews 2013*, (6). DOI: 10.1002/14651858.CD003260. pub2. www. cochranelibrary.com.

Barnes, D. E., Santos-Modesitt, W., Poelke, G., Kramer, A. F., Castro, C., Middleton, L. E. et al. (2013). The Mental Activity and eXercise (MAX) trial: A randomized controlled trial to enhance cognitive function in older adults. *JAMA Internal Medicine*, 173 (9), 797–804.

Bateman, D. R., Srinivas, B., Emmett, T. W., Schleyer, T. K., Holden, R. J., Hendrie., H. C. et al. (2017). Categorizing health outcomes and efficacy of mHealth apps for persons with cognitive impairment: A systematic review. *Journal of Medical Internet Research*, 19 (8), 3301.

Blattgerste, J., Renner, P., & Pfeiffer, T. (2019). Augmented reality action assistance and learning for cognitively impaired people: A systematic literature review. *PETRA '19: Proceedings of the 12th ACM International Conference on Pervasive Technologies Related to Assistive Environments*, 270–279. https://doi.org/10.1145/3316782.3316789.

Bonini, M. V. & Mansur, L. L. (2009). Comprehension and storage of radio news items: Comprehension and storage of sequentially presented radio news items by healthy elderly. *Dementia & Neuropsychologia*, 3 (2), 118–123.

Bourgeois, M. S. (1992). Evaluating memory wallets in conversations with patients with dementia. *Journal of Speech and Hearing Research*, 35 (6), 1344–1357.

Bourgeois. M. S. (2014). *Memory and communication aids for people with dementia*. Health Professions Press Inc. Boltimore.

Bourgeois, M. S., Burgio, L. D., Schulz, R., Beach, S., & Palmer, B. (1997). Modifying repetitive verbalizations of community-dwelling patients with AD. *The Cerontologist*, 37 (1), 30–39.

Burgio, L., Allen-Burge, R., Roth, D., Bourgeois, M., Dijkstra, K., Gerstle, J., Jackson, E., & Bankester, L. (2001). Come talk with me: Improving communication between nursing assistants and nursing home residents during care routines. *The Gerontologist*, 41, 449–460.

Busse, A., Hensel, A., Gühne, U., Angermeyer, M. C., & Riedel-Heller, S. G. (2006). Mild cognitive impairment. Long-term course of four clinical Subtypes. *Neurology*, 67, 2176–2185.

Cheung, G. & Peri, K. (2021). Challenges to dementia care during COVID-19: Innovations in remote delivery of group Cognitive Stimulation Therapy. *Aging & Mental Health*, 25 (6), 977–979, DOI: 10.1080/13607863.2020.1789945.

Dahlke, D. V. & Ory, M. G. (2020). Emerging issues of intelligent assistive technology use among people with dementia and their caregivers: A U.S. perspective. *Frontiers Public Health*, https://doi.org/10.3389/fpubh.2020.00191.

D'Cunha, N. M., Nguyen, D., Naumovski, N., McKune, A. J., Kellett, J., Georgousopoulou, E. N. et al. (2019). Mini-review of virtual reality-based interventions to promote well-being for people living with dementia and mild cognitive impairment. *Gerontology*, 65, 430–440, DOI: 10.1159/000500040.

Doi, T., Kuwahara, N., & Morimoto, K. (2016). Assessing the use of communication robots for recreational activities at nursing homes based on dementia care mapping (DCM). Duffy, V. G. (Ed.). *Digital human modeling: Applications in health, safety, ergonomics and risk management*. Springer. pp. 203–211.

Drucker, P. F. (2012). *Innovation and entrepreneurship*. Routledge.

Ferreira, L. D. A., Ferreira, H., Cavaco, S., Cameirão, M., & Badia, S. B. (2020). User experience of interactive technologies for people with dementia: Comparative observational study. *JMIR Serious Games 2020*, 8 (3), e17565, doi: 10.2196/17565.

Folstein, M. F., Folstein, S. E., & Mchugh, P. R. (1975). Mini-mental state: A practical method for grading the cognitive state of patients for the clinician. *Journal of Psychiatric Research*, 12, 189–198.

Flores, S., Bailey, H. R., Eisenberg, M. L., & Zacks, J. M. (2017). Event segmentation improves event memory up to one month later. *Journal of Experimental Psychology: Learning, Memory, and Cognition*, 43 (8), 1183–1202. https://doi.org/10.1037/xlm0000367.

Foster, B. (2009). Music for life's journey: The capacity of music in dementia care. *Alzheimer's Care Today*. 10 (1), 42–49. Doi.10.1097/ACQ.0b013e3181974684.

Fujita, I. (2009). *Nou boom no meishin* [Superstition about the brain boom]. Asukashinsha. (in Japanese)

Fujita, I. & Abe, M. (Eds.) (2009). *Koji nou kinoushougai gaku* [Higher brain dysfunction]. Igakushoin. (in Japanese)

Gottfries, C. G., Bråne, G., Gullberg, B., & Steen, G. (1982). A new rating scale for dementia syndromes. *Archives of Gerontology and Geriatrics*, 1 (4), 311–330.

Gowans, G., Campbell, J., Alm, A., Dye, R., Astell, A., & Ellid, M. (2004). Designing a multimedia conversation aid for reminiscence therapy in dementia care environments. *CHI 2004 Conference on Human Factors in Computing Systems*, 825–836, https://doi.org/10.1145/985921.985943.

Greenaway, M. C., Duncan, N. L., & Smith, G. E. (2013). The memory support system for mild cognitive impairment: Randomized trial of cognitive rehabilitation intervention. *International Journal of Geriatric Psychiatry*, 28 (4), 402–409.

Grossi, F., Bianchi, V., Matrella, G., de Munari, I., & Ciampolini, P. (2014). Senior-friendly kitchen activity: The FOOD Project. *Gerontechnology*, 13 (2), 200–200. https://doi.org/10.4017/gt.2014.13.02.349.00.

Helmes, E., Csapo, K. G., & Short, J. (1987), A. Standardization and Validation of the Multidimensional Observation Scale for Elderly Subjects (MOSES), *Journal of Gerontology*, 42 (4), 395–405. https://doi.org/10.1093/geronj/42.4.395.

Hickey, E. M. & Bourgeois, M. S. (2018). Cognitive and communicative interventions. 168–213. in E. Hickey & M. Bourgeois (Eds.) *Dementia: Person-centered assessment and intervention (2nd Ed.)*. New York: Taylor & Francis.

Hickey, E. M., Bourgeois, M. S., & Brush, J. (2018). Interprofessional interventions for participation and quality of life. 214–259. in E. Hickey & M. Bourgeois (Eds.) *Dementia: Person-centered assessment and intervention (2nd Ed.)*. New York: Taylor & Francis.

Hickey, M., Khayum, B., & Bourgeois, M. S. (2018). Assessment of cognition, communication, and behavior. *Dementia: Person-centered assessment and intervention (2nd Ed.)*. New York: Taylor & Francis. 113–167.

Honma, A., Yatomi, T., & Shigeta, M. (2008). *Ninchishou no yobou/shien manual.* [Prevention and support manual for dementia]. http://www.tmig.or.jp/kaigoyobou/08_ninchishou.pdf. (In Japanese)

Hopper, T., Hickey, E. M., & Bourgeois, M. S. (2018). Clinical and pathophysiological, profiles of various dementia etiologies. 11-41. in E. Hickey & M. Bourgeois (Eds.) *Dementia: Person-centered assessment and intervention*. New York: Taylor & Francis.

Ienca, M,, Fabrice, J., Elger, B., Caon, M., Pappagallo, A. S., Kressig, R. W. et al. (2017). Intelligent assistive technology for Alzheimer's disease and other dementias: A systematic review. *Journal of Alzheimer's Disease*, 56 (4), 1301–1340, DOI: 10.3233/JAD-161037.

Ikota, T. (2016). *Yonshussaikarano ninchishou yobou nyumon* [Introduction to dementia prevention from the age of 40]. Koudansha Blue Backs. (in Japanese)

Ingram, A. (2012) Critical Review: Does music therapy have a positive impact on language functioning in adults with dementia? *Reviews Western University Canada 2012: 2011–12.*

Irazoki, E., Contreras-Somoza, L. M., Toribio-Guzmán, J. M., Jenaro-Río, C., van der Roest, H., & Franco-Martín, M. A. (2020). Technologies for cognitive training and cognitive rehabilitation for people with mild cognitive impairment and dementia: A systematic review. *Frontiers in Psychology*, 11, https://www.frontiersin.org/article/10.3389/fpsyg.2020.00648, DOI: 10.3389/fpsyg.2020.00648.

Japanese Society of Neurology (2012). *Ninchisho shikkan shinryou guideline* [Practice guidelines for dementia disease] *2010: Compact ban 2012.* Igakushoin. (in Japanese)

Japanese Society of Neurology (2017). *Ninchisho shikkann shinryou guideline 2017* [Practice guidelines for dementia disease 2017]. Igakushoin. (in Japanese)

Japan Society for Dementia Prevention (2013). *Ninchisho yobou senmonshi textbook* [Dementia prevention specialist textbook]. Tokuma Shoten. (in Japanese)

Japan Society for Higher Brain Dysfunction (2014). *Standard verbal paired-associate learning test.* Shinkoh Igaku Shuppansha. (in Japanese)

Kaneko, M. (1990). Chihoto zentoyokino [Dementia and frontal lobe function]. *Shitsugosyo Kenkyu* [Higher Brain Function Research], 10 (2), 127–131. https://doi.org/10.2496/apr.10.127. (In Japanese)

Karasawa, H., Yasuma, Y., & Udagawa, M. (2014). Monowasure speed monshinhyou [Forgetfulness speed questionnaire]. *Gekkan Tiiki Igaku* [Monthly Community Medicine], 6, 504–512. (in Japanese)

Kawashima, R. (2003a). *Koujinou no brain imaging* [Brain imaging of higher brain function]. Igaku-shoin. p. 91. (In Japanese)

Kawato, S., Utsumi, A., & Abe, S. (2006). Gaze direction estimation with a single camera based on four reference points and three calibration images. *Asian Conference on Computer Vision (ACCV 20069).* 419–428.

Kazui, H., Sato, S., Yoshiyama, K., & Kanemoto, H. (2020). Success rate of various countermeasures against behavioral psychological symptoms of dementia based on the accumulation of real-world experience. *International Psychogeriatrics*, 32, S1, P115, 2020.

Kiyohara, Y. (2014). *Wagakuni niokeru koureisha ninchishou no jittai to taisaku* [Actual situations and countermeasures for elderly dementia in Japan]. October 19, 2014. http://www.kantei.go.jp/jp/singi/kenkouiryou/suisin/suisin_dai4/siryou7.pdf. (In Japanese)

Kosugi, N., Sato, S., Yoshiyama, K., Noguchi, D., Yamanaka, K., & Kazui, H. (2020). *Ninchisho chienowa-net*: A web system that calculates and publishes the probability of success of coping methods for behavioral and psychological symptoms of dementia. *iiWAS '20 (Information Integration and Web-based Applications*

& Services 2020). 383–389. https://doi.org/10.1145/3428757.3429119.

Koutentakis, D., Pilozzi, A., & Huang, X. (2020). Designing socially assistive robots for Alzheimer's disease and related dementia patients and their caregivers: Where we are and where we are headed. *Healthcare*, 8, 73, DOI: 10.3390/healthcare8020073.

Kuwahara, N., Kuwabara, K., Tetsutani, S., & Yasuda, K. (2005). Reminiscence video: Helping at-home caregivers of people with people with Dementia. A. Sloane (Ed.) *Home-Oriented Informatics and Telematics*. Springer, pp. 145–154.

Kuwahara, N., Kuwabara, K., Utsumi, A., Yasuda, K., & Tetsutani, N. (2004). Networked interaction therapy: Relieving stress in memory-impaired people and their family mmbers. *The 26th Annual International Conference of the IEEE Engineering in Medicine and Biology Society.* https://ieeexplore.ieee.org/abstract/document/1403886/citations?tabFilter=papers.

Kuwahara, N., Yasuda, K., Tetsutani, N., & Moromoto, K. (2010). Remote assistance for people with dementia at home using reminiscence systems and a schedule prompter. *International Journal of Computers in Healthcare*. Springer. pp. 126–143.

Livingston, G., Sommerlad, A., Orteta, V., Costafreda, S., Huntley, J., Ames, D. et al. (2017). Dementia prevention, intervention, and care. *The Lancet Commissions July 20.* http://dx.doi.org/10.1016/S0140-6736(17)31363-6

Lund, D. A., Hill, R. D., Caserta, M. S., & Wright, S. D.(1995). Video respite TM: An innovative resource for family, professional caregivers, and persons with dementia. *The Gerontologist*, 35, 683–687.

Maeda, H., Saiki, S., Nakamura, M., & Yasuda, K. (2019). Memory aid service using mind sensing and daily retrospective by virtual agent. *HCI International*, LNCS 11582 (2), 353–364.

Mahendra, N. (2001). Direct intervention for improving the performance of individuals with alzheimer's disease. *Seminars in Speech & Language*, 22 (4), 289–302.

Mahendra, N., Hickey, E. M., & Bourgeois, M. S. (2018). Cognitive-communicative characteristics: Profiling types of dementia. 42-80P, in E. Hickey & M. Bourgeois (Eds.) (2018). *Dementia: Person-centered assessment and intervention.* New York: Taylor & Francis.

Matsuda, H. (2016). MRI morphometry in Alzheimer's disease. *Ageing Research Reviews*, 30, 17–24. https://doi.org/10.1016/j.arr.2016.01.003.

Matsuda, O. (2017). Koureishano chitekikatudoto sono eikyo [Intellectual activity and its effects among older people]. *Rounen Seishin Igaku Zasshi* [Japanese Journal of Geriatric Psychiatry], 28 (1), 11–18. (in Japanese)

McDermott, O., Crellin, N., Ridder, H. M., & Orrell, M. (2012). Music therapy in dementia: A narrative synthesis systematic review. *International Journal of geriatric Psychiatry*. https://doi.org/10.1002/gps.3895.

McKhann, G. M., Knopman, D. S., Chertkow, H., Hyman, B. T., Jack Jr, C. R. et al. (2011). The diagnosis of dementia due to Alzheimer's disease: Recommendations from the National Institute on Aging-Alzheimer's Association workgroups on diagnostic guidelines for Alzheimer's disease. *Alzheimer's and*

Dementia, 7, 263–269. https://doi.org/10.1016/j.jalz.2011.03.005.

Meiland, F., Innes, A., Mountain, G., Robinson, L., van der Roest, H., García-Casal, J. A. (2017). Technologies to support community-dwelling persons with dementia: A position paper on issued regarding development, usability, effectiveness and cost-effectiveness, deployment, and ethics. *JMIR Rehabilitation Assistive Technologies*, 4 (1). http://rehab.jmir.org.

Meyers, J. E. & Meyers, K. R. (1995). Rey complex figure test under four different administration procedures. *The Clinical Neuropsychologist*, 9 (1). 63–67. https://doi.org/10.1080/13854049508402059.

Miura, C., Saiki, S., Nakamura, M., & Yasuda, K. (2020). Implementing and evaluating feedback feature of mind monitoring service for elderly people at home. *International Conference on Information Integration and Web-based Applications & Services (iiWAS2020)*, 390–395.

Mulvenna, M. D. & Nugent, C. D. (Eds.) (2010). *Supporting people with dementia using pervasive health technologies*. Springer. London.

Nakagawa, Y. & Obo, I. (1985). *Nihonban GHQ seishin kenko thousahyou tebiki* [Japanese version of GHQ Mental Health Questionnaire Guide]. Nihon Bunka Kagakusha. (in Japanese)

Nakajima, M., Ebihara, N., Saijo, T., & Ohira, H. (2013). Ongakuno sutoresu kaisyou koukani tsuite [The effect of music on stress relief]. *Ningen Kankyougaku Kennkyuu* [Journal of Human Environmental Studies], 11 (1), 19–25. (in Japanese)

Nakatani, S., Saiki, S., Nakamura, M., & Yasuda, K. (2018). Generating personalized virtual agent in speech dialogue system for people with dementia. *HCI International 2018*, LNCS 10917, 326-337.

Nakayama, K., Hara, T., & Nishio, S. (2006). Wikipedia mining niyoru sisorasujisyono koutikusyuhou [Wikipedia Mining to Construct a Thesaurus]. *IPSJ Journal*, 47 (10), 2917–2928. (in Japanese)

Narumoto, J. (2016). *Ninnchisyono hitono iryousenntakuto ishikettei sienn* [Medical selection and decision support for people with dementia]. Creates Kamogawa. (in Japanese)

Narumoto, J. (Ed.) (2017). *Jissen, Ninchisyono hitoni yasashii kinnyu gaido* [Practical guide for dementia friendly financial services]. Creates Kamogawa. (in Japanese)

New Orange Plan (2015). https://www.mhlw.go.jp/english/policy/care-welfare/care-welfare-elderly/dl/ltcisj_e.pdf.

NIH (2019–2020). Behavioral and Lifestyle Interventions for Prevention and treatment. https://www.nia.nih.gov/report-2019-2020-scientific-advances-prevention-treatment-and-care-dementia/behavioral-and??.

Onoda, K. & Yamaguchi, S. (2014). *Ninchisho masusukuri-ninngu niokeru aipadno ouyou* [Utilization of iPad for Dementia Mass Screening: CADi Development and Verification]. *Plos One*. https://doi.org/10.1371/journal.pone.0109931. (in Japanese)

Oshima, C., Itou, N., Nishimoto, K., Yasuda, K., Hosoi, N., Yamashita, H. et al. (2013). A music therapy system for patients with dementia who repeat stereotypical utterances. *Journal of Information Processing*, 21 (2), 283–294.

Oshima, C., Yasuda, K., Uno, T., Machishima, K., & Nakayama, K. (2015). Give a dog ICT devices: How smartphone-carrying assistance dogs may help people with dementia. *International Journal of Advanced Computer Science and Applications*, 6 (1), 168–176.

Otake, M. (2012). *Kaigo ni yakudatu kyousouhou* [Co-reminiscent therapy for efficient care]. Chuohoki Publishing. (in Japanese)

Ougizawa, N. (2015). Ninchisho honnin totomoni kangaeru seikatsushougai heno approach [Considering the approaches to daily life disability with dementia patients]. *Japanese Journal of Geriatric Psychiatry*, 26 (9), 973–981. (in Japanese)

Owen, A. M., Hampshire, A., Grahn, J. A., Stenton, R., Dajani, S., Burns, A. S et al. (2010). Putting brain training to the test. *Nature*, 465, 775–778.

Ozono, H., Chen, S., & Nakamura, M. (2021). Study of microservice execution framework using spoken dialogue agents. *IEEE-ACIS International Conference on Software Engineering, Artificial Intelligence, Networking and Parallel Distributed Computing (SNPD2021)*, Nov. 2021. (in press)

Petersen, R. C., Smith, G. E., Waring, S. C., Ivnik, R. J., Tangalos, E. G., & Kokmen, E. (1999). Mild cognitive impairment: Clinical characterization and outcome. *Arch Neurol*, 56 (3), 303–308.

Riyan, E., Tanimoto, T., Sano, M., & Yasuda, K. (2017). Hitodousa ninshiki oyobi buttaininshiki womochiita okiwasure shien [Misplacement-prevention support using human motion recognition and object recognition]. *IPSJ SIG Technical Reports. ASD.* 2017-ASD-7 (3), 1–5. IPSJ-ASD17007003.pdf. (in Japanese)

Sakai, Y., Nonaka, Y., Yasuda, K., & Nakano, Y. I. (2012). Listener agent for elderly people with dementia. *Proceedings of the seventh annual ACM/IEEE international conference on Human-Robot Interaction (HRI2012)*. 199–200.

Salthouse, T. A., Mitchell, D. R., Skovronek, E., Babcock, R. L. et al., (1989). Effects of adult age and working memory on reasoning and spatial abilities. *Journal of Experimental Psychology; Learning, Memory and Cognition*, 15, 507–516.

Sano, M., Miyawaki, K., Mitsumori, H., Ohtani, K., Yoneyama, S., & Ohde, M. (2013). Remote cognitive rehabilitation support system for menu and meal preparation. *CEA '13: Proceedings of the 5th international workshop on Multimedia for cooking & eating activities*, 27–32. https://doi.org/10.1145/2506023.2506029.

Sohlberg, M. M. & Mateer, C. A. (1989). Training use of compensatory memory books: A three-stage behavioral approach. *Journal of Clinical and Experimental Neuro Psychology*, 11 (6), 871–891.

Sone, D., Imabayashi, Maikusa, E., Ogawa, M., Sato, N., & Matsuda, H. (2018). Voxel-based specific regional analysis system for Alzheimer's disease (VSRAD) on 3-tesla normal database: Diagnostic accuracy in two independent cohorts with early Alzheimer's disease. *Aging Disease*, 9 (4), 755–760. doi: 10.14336/AD.2017.0818.

Srisamosorn, N., Kuwahara, N., Yamashita, A., Ogata, T., & Ota, J (2016). Design of face tracking system using fixed 360 degree cameras and flying blimp for health care evaluation. *Proceedings of the 4th International Conference on Serviceology (ICSery, 2016)*, 63–66.

Standard Language Test of Aphasia (SLTA, 1977). *Hyoujyun shitsugoshou kensa tebiki* [Manual of Standard Language Test of Aphasia], Houmeido. (In Japanese)

Takase, Y., Yoshida, Y., Dohi, S., Nakano, I, C., Sakai, N., & Yasuda, K. (2016). Animation agent tono doukou toshita hokou training system no teian [A system supporting walking exercise through strolling with a companion agent]. *The 30th Annual Conference of the Japanese Society for Artificial Intelligence.* https://www.ai-gakkai.or.jp/jsai2016/webprogram/2016/pdf/615.pdf. (in Japanese)

Tamamizu, K., Sakakibara, S., Saiki, S., Nakamura, M., & Yasuda, K. (2017). Capturing activities of daily living for elderly at home based on environment change and speech dialog. *Digital Human Modeling 2017*, LNCS 10287, 183–194.

Tokunaga, S., Tamamizu, K., Saiki, S., Nakamura, M., & Yasuda, K. (2016). Virtual CareGiver: Personalized smart elderly care. *International Journal of Software Innovation*, 5 (1), 30–43.

Utsumi, A., Kanbara, D., Kawato, S., Abe, S., & Yamauchi, H. (2006). Vison-based detention for monitoring and assisting memory-impaired people. *International Workshop on Cognitive Prostheses and Assisted Communication (CPAC 2006)*, 10–15.

Wechsler, D. (1997). *Wecheler memory scale-reviced.* Translated by Sugishita, 2001. Nihon Bunka Kagakusha. (in Japanese)

Welland, R. J., Lubinski, R., & Higginbotham, D. J. (2002). Discourse Comprehension Test: Performance of elders with dementia of the Alzheimer type. *Journal of Speech, Language, and Hearing Research*, 45 (6), 1175–1187.

Yamaguchi, H. (2010). *Ninchisho no tadashii rikai to houkatsuteki iryou, care no point* [Correct understanding of dementia and points of comprehensive medicine and care], 2nd ed. Kyodo Isho Shuppan. (in Japanese)

Yamashita, H. (2007). Honpou seijinnniokeru Rey-Osterrieth hukuzatsu zukeino kijyun de-ta [A normative study of Rey-Osterrieth complex figure in normal Japanese adults]. *Clinical Psychiatry*, 49 (2), 155–159. (in Japanese)

Yamazaki, M. (2008–2009). Hito, mono, ba wo tsunagu ninchishou care [Dementia care that connects people, things, and fields]. *Houmonkango to kaigo* (serialization), 13 (7)–14 (9). Igaku-shoin. (In Japanese)

Yamazaki, M. (2015). *Rounen design gaku* [Geriatric design studies]. *Fukushikaigo Techno Plus*, 1, 22–27. (in Japanese)

Yasuda, K., Okada, T., Sadohara, M., Yoshitake, N., Uchimura, H., & Ono, Y. (1993). Shougaisya gallery rehabili bijyutukan; asuheno madono innai secchito QOL [Rehabilitation museum: Window toward tomorrow-institution of gallery for the disabled in the hospital and QOL]. *Sogo Rehabilitation*, 21 (11), 977–980. (in Japanese)

Yasuda, K., Watanabe, O., & Ono, Y. (1997). Dissociation between semantic and autobiographic memory: A case report. *Cortex*, 33 (4), 623–638.

Yasuda, K. & Ono, Y. (1998). Comprehension of famous personal and geographical names in global aphasic subjects. *Brain and Language*, 61 (2), 274–287.

Yasuda, K., Misu, T., Murasugi, K., Miyazaki, T., & Nakamura, T. (1999). Zenkukenbou tou no shien wo mokutekitoshita onsei shutsuryoku kioku hojyoki no kaihatu [Development of voice output memory aid for supporting anterograde amnesia]. *Sogo Rehabilitation*, 27 (5), 475–478. (in Japanese)

Yasuda, K., Nakamura, T., & Beckma, B. (2000a). Brain processing of proper names. *Aphasiology*, 14 (11), 1067–1090.

Yasuda, K. & Nakamura, T. (2000b). Comprehension of serially presented radio news story. *Brain and Language*, 75 (3), 399–415.

Yasuda, K., Misu, T., Beckman, B., Watanabe, O., Ozawa, Y., & Nakamura, T. (2002a). Use of IC recorder as a voice output memory aid for patients with prospective memory impairment. *Neuropsychological Rehabilitation*, 12 (2), 155–156.

Yasuda, K., Misu, T., Iwamoto, A., & Nakamura, T. (2002b). Denshikikiniyoru onseiyudode mondaikodoga genshoshita Alzheimer's disease no ichirei [Successful use of voice output navigator for a patient with Alzheimer's disease]. *Higher Brain Function Research*, 22, 292–299. (in Japanese)

Yasuda, K. (2003a). *Shitsugoshousha no danwa to koyumeishi no rikai* [Comprehension of discourse and proper names people with aphasia] (Doctoral thesis). https://gensoshi.jimdofree.com/english-home-page/. (in Japanese)

Yasuda, K., Iwamoto, A., & Nakamura, T. (2003b). Kimeiryoku shougaisha eno soukishien [Retrieval support for people with memory disabilities]. *Shitsugosyo Kenkyu* [Higher Brain Function Research], 23, 60–61. (in Japanese)

Yasuda, K., Beckman, B., Yoneda, M., Toneda, H., Iwamoto, A., & Nakamura, T. (2006a). Successful guidance by automatic output of music and verbal messages for daily behavioral disturbances of three individuals with dementia. *Neuropsychological Rehabilitation*, 16 (1), 66–82.

Yasuda, K. (2007a). Keitaidenwa wo mochiita kiokushien [Memory support using mobile phones]. *Houmonkango to Kaigo* [The Japanese Journal of Home Care Nursing], 12 (11), 944–949. (in Japanese).

Yasuda, K., Nemoto, T., Takenaka, K., Mitach, M., & Kuwabara, K. (2007b). Effectiveness of vocabulary data file, encyclopedia, and Internet homepages in a conversation support system for people with moderate-severe aphasia. *Aphasiology*, 21 (9), 867–882.

Yasuda, K. (2007c). Rehabilitation through portable and electronic memory aids at different stages of Alzheimer's disease. *Les Cahiers De La Fondation Me'de'ric Alzheimer*, 3, 97–107.

Yasuda, K. (2008a). Kougakuteki shienkenkyu no saizensen [Forefront of engineering support research for dementia]. *Houmonkango to Kaigo*, [The Japanese Journal of Home Care Nursing], 13 (3), 234–239. (in Japanese)

Yasuda, K. (2008b). Asuno egao wo shinjiyo [Believe in tomorrow's smile]. *Houmonkango to Kaigo* [The Japanese Journal of Home Care Nursing], 13 (4), 324–328. (in Japanese)

Yasuda, K., Okazaki, Y., Utsumi, A., Yamazoe, H., & Abe, S. (2008c). Ninchisho muke toire dousa shien system shisaku: Toire mogikankyo deno hyouka [Toilet-steps support system prototype for dementia: Evaluation in a toilet simulation environment]. *Higher Brain Function Research*, 29 (1), 178–179. (in Japanese)

Yasuda, K., Kuwabara, K., Kuwahara, N., Abe, S., & Tetsutani, N. (2009). Effectiveness of personalized reminiscence photo videos for individuals with dementia. *Neuropsychological Rehabilitation*, 19 (4), 603–619.

Yasuda, K., Namakura, M., kuwahara, N., Nakamura, T., & Iwamoto, A. (2011). Kogata bideoki to onseininshiki niyoru koudoukiroku kensakushistemu no kaihatsu [Development of behavior's records & searching system by small video devise and voice recognition]. *Higher Brain Function Research*, 31 (1), 86–87. (in Japanese)

Yasuda, K., Kuwahara, N., Nakamura, M., Morimoto, K., Nakayama, K., Oshima, C., & Aoe, J. (2012). Assistance dogs for individuals with dementia using ICT devices: Proposal of human-computer-animal interface, ICHS (International Conference of Humanized Systems), ICHS CD-Rom, OS01_1010.

Yasuda, K. (2013a). *Shin kioku sapoto cho* [New memory support diary]. ESCOR. (in Japanese).

Yasuda, K., Kuwahara, N., Kuwabara, K., Morimoto, K., & Tetsutani, N. (2013b). Daily assistance for individuals with dementia via video phone. *American Journal of Alzheimer's Disease & Other Dementias*, 28 (5), 508–516.

Yasuda, K., Aoe, J., & Fuketa, M. (2013). Development of an agent system for conversing with individuals with dementia. *The Japanese Society for Artificial Intelligence*, https://doi.org/10.11517/pjsai.JSAI2013.0_3C1IOS1b2.

Yasuda, K., Fuketa, M., Morita, K., Aoe, J., & Kuwahara, M. (2016b). Video phone conversation of two individuals with dementia using an anime agent system. *Lecture Notes in Computer Science (LNCS)*, 9745. 317–326. Springer Publishing.

Yasuda, K., Narumoto, J., Sano, M., Kuwahara, N., & Kuwabara, K. (2019). The sustained and selective effectiveness of a videophone conversation for individuals with dementia. *Journal of Alzheimer's Research and Therapy*, 1 (1), 6–14.

Yokoi, K., Nishio, Y., Uchiyama, M., Shimomura, T., & Iizuka, O. (2014). Hallucinators find meaning in noises: Pareidolic illusions in dementia with lewy bodies. *Neuropsychologia*, 56, 245–254.

Yoneyama, K. (2010). *Ninchisho wa yobo dekiru* [Dementia can be prevented]. Chikumashobo. (in Japanese)

Relevant books

Astell, A., Smith, S. K., & Joddrell, P. (Eds.) (2019). *Using technology in dementia care*. London and Philadelphia; Jessica Kingsley Publishers.

Hickey, E. & Bourgeois, M. (Eds.) (2018). *Dementia: Person-centered assessment and intervention (2nd Ed.)*. New York: Taylor & Francis.

Jotterand, F., Ienca, M., & Wangmo, T. (Eds.) (2019). *Intelligent assistive technologies for dementia: Clinical, ethical, social, and regulatory implications*. New York; Oxford University Press.

Mulvenna, M. D. & Nugent, C. D. (Eds.) (2010). *Supporting people with dementia using pervasive health technologies*. London. Springer.

Sixsmith, A., Sixsmith, J., Fang, M. L., & Horst, B. (2020). *AgeTech, cognitive health, and dementia: Synthesis lectures on assistive, rehabilitative, and health-preserving technologies*. Morgan & Claypool Publishers.

Appendix

Appendix 1

Form for detecting MCI/dementia (for barbers/hairdressers) (draft)
Items to check

		Date checked Month/Date		
1.	Clothes are not sensible for the season.	/	/	/
2.	The customer's visits for a haircut have become irregular.	/	/	/
3.	The customer looks less motivated and says that she/he wishes to do nothing.	/	/	/
4.	The customer shows ups and downs in emotions.	/	/	/
5.	The customer talks about the same things repeatedly.	/	/	/
6.	In paying and counting change, the customer shows some confusion.	/	/	/
7.	In front of the shop, when the customer happens to pass by, we greet her/him by calling her/his name, yet, she/he walks away without responding.	/	/	/
8.		/	/	/
9.		/	/	/
10.		/	/	/

(Other behaviors you are concerned about) ______________________

____

If your customer has many of the behaviors on this form, please talk to the customer and suggest that the customer's family members contact regional comprehensive support centers.

Eight types of forms are currently available: for using at shops, at banks, at pharmacies, at dentists/hospitals, at barbers/hairdressers, at social clubs, at delivery services, and in neighborhoods. You can download them from the following website (https://gensoshi.jimdofree.com/home-pages-for-english/ or, search "Kiyoshi Yasuda homepage").

by Kiyoshi Yasuda, June 24, 2021

Appendix 2

Consent form on mutual surveillance for MCI/dementia and helping each other (draft)

Date: ______________

MCI/dementia is a disease often seen among elderly people. The main symptom is forgetfulness. As the disease usually develops over several years, people are not often conscious of the symptoms. Some people tend to deny their forgetfulness if they are told by their family members, which often makes it difficult to detect and deal with the problems at an early stage. Several medicines for preventing the progress of forgetfulness are now prescribed, though the effectiveness of the medicines are still limited.

Therefore, we now make a promise about the following matters. We, as good friends, will watch out for forgetfulness in each other. If we detect worsening forgetfulness in one of us, we will recommend the friend take proper action, such as going to see a doctor at a memory clinic.

Even if our friends are diagnosed with MCI/dementia, we promise to continue helping each other.

Name ____________ Sign Date ____________ Tel. ____________
Address ____
My wishes: ____
____

Name ____________ Sign Date ____________ Tel. ____________
Address ____
My wishes ____
____

Name ____________ Sign Date ____________ Tel. ____________
Address ____
My wishes ____
____

by Kiyoshi Yasuda, June 24, 2021

Appendix 3

Dementia declaration and request form for assistance (draft)

Date: ______________

To Whom It May Concern:

Name __________________

I hereby declare that I have dementia. Dementia is a disease with memory impairment and other cognitive dysfunction. Since around the year _______, I have been suffering from the disease which causes me to forget what I have heard, how to use devices and operate electric appliances, the faces of the persons I have met, and other important things.

I might become disoriented in dates/locations and may ask the same questions repeatedly.

Around _______________, I was diagnosed as having dementia.

Today, I have the following difficulties:

I will continue trying to avoid trouble. However, when I have problems, please give me your support as follows:

Name ____
Address ____
Contact no. ____

Family member ____
Address ____
Contact no. ____

Family member ____
Address ____
Contact no. ____

by Kiyoshi Yasuda, June 24, 2021

Appendix 4

Summarized list of memory strategies for the healthy elderly

Let's prepare for having MCI/dementia and the end of life.

by Kiyoshi Yasuda, June 24, 2021

1. To prepare for the end of your life, first, write statements of your will in the ending note. You should write your wishes for the possibility that you become bedridden and/or need life-prolonging treatments.
2. To prevent fires, change your cooking system to an IH stove, and install sensors and an alarm system for heat, gas, and smoke in the house.
3. Use the New Memory Support Diary, or the Diary *Tomorrow* to reduce the frequency of forgetfulness (see Yasuda, 2022 *). The diary should be left open on your desk so that you can write in it immediately information that you want to remember at a later time. Share the diary with your family members who may write in the diary with a pen in a different color. In this way, the diary can serve as a message board among the family members.
4. Use memo-pads or make a wearable memo-pad with sticky-notes (see Yasuda's website *). Carry it all the time and write down whatever you want to remember before you forget. Then, paste the sticky-notes into the Memory Support Diary to review later.
5. If you own many personal belongings, organize them and keep them in a special location. This may prevent you from misplacing them and will take less time to look for them.
6. Decide on a location to keep your bankbooks and other valuables. In spite of that, if you often misplace them, ask your children to take care of them for you. For other daily-use objects, you may place them in transparent boxes at the entrance to your house or in your room. You can also use wall hangings with transparent pockets. Attach a name tag to each pocket to show what is in there.
7. Record messages for taking medicines and other daily routines on the Sony IC Recorder (ICD-PX240, about 50 dollars). Then, set times and dates for the messages to be emitted from the device. Once you set them, the recorded messages are output automatically.
8. Use the alarm function of a smartphone to remind you of the time to take your medicines, for example. If the GPS function is installed, your family members can locate you in case you have an accident or if you

get lost. You should be familiar with using your smartphone before your memory deteriorates.

9. You can use electronic medicine boxes that have a timer to set an alarm for taking medicine at specific times.
10. Start having conversations with your friends and relatives using a videophone on your smartphone or PC (e.g., Skype, Zoom, LINE). It is recommended to set up a conversation club to develop networks for remote mutual support.
11. Wear a vest with many pockets, and put your glasses, memo-pads, etc. in the pockets. Cargo pants and skirts with multiple pockets are also convenient. Decide what you put in a particular pocket. By touching the surface of these pockets, you can confirm what is in them.
12. When you are told to stop driving by your doctor, friends, or family members, consider using public transportation systems, a powered bicycle, an electric scooter, or a nursing-care taxi. You should realize that the laws regulating drivers with dementia are becoming more strict.
13. Organize your photo albums and put titles on each photo. The photos with titles will be useful for stimulating your memory when you have dementia.
14. Learn about the nursing care insurance program and methods for caring for the elderly. In order to learn them, attend peer group meetings for family members. You may also go to elderly facilities as a volunteer worker. It is a good opportunity to consider what kind of care and facility will be good for you if you have to receive nursing care.
15. Decide on your legal guardian. Consult with your guardian as well as your banks, trust companies, and other insurance companies for managing your money and your property. You may also contact the social welfare council in your area about the adult guardianship system.
16. Store various ID's and passwords for digital properties (cards, devices, onlines, etc.) in one place. Give a copy to a family member.

* Kiyoshi Yasuda (2022). *Rehabilitation for MCI and Dementia: Using Assistive Technology to Support Daily Activities*, published by Union Press. See the following website of Kiyoshi Yasuda: https://gensoshi.jimdofree.com/home-pages-for-english/, or search with "Kiyoshi Yasuda homepage."

Appendix 5

Detailed list of memory strategies for the healthy elderly

Let's prepare for having MCI/dementia and the end of life.

by Kiyoshi Yasuda, June 24, 2021

Table of contents

1. How should I manage my belongings?

- The more you have, the more you have to look for. Dispose of unneeded belongings by giving them to others or selling them at bazaars.
- Use hanging transparent pockets and paste labels on the pockets. After coming home, change your clothes beside the hanging pockets in order to put the belongings into the pockets immediately after taking them from your clothes.
- Place your glasses and other belongings in a transparent box on the desk. Do not keep the box inside a drawer; this makes it difficult for you to confirm whether all the objects are there.
- Use only one bag if possible. Or, decide to use one bag for each destination, such as one for hospitals or shopping. Then, decide what to put in each bag.
- A cross-body bag is better than a handbag to prevent you from leaving it behind. Attach your name and a contact number tag to your bag.
- Wear a vest with many pockets and decide what to put in the pockets. If you find it too heavy for your shoulders, wear a pair of cargo pants with many pockets which reduces the burden on your shoulders.
- Attach stretchable or spring-like cords to your wallet, pass cases, etc. Then, attach a colored clip at the end of each cord, and connect the clip to your pockets or bags. Use different color clips for different objects, so that you will know which are tied to which. You can pull the cord when

you look for an object. You may attach a cord also to your bag and tie it to your clothes with the cord so as not to leave the bag behind.

- When you do gardening, wrap fluorescent or luminescence tapes around gardening tools. By this way, they are easy to see after dark.
- Buy GPS sets for locating lost objects. The set consists of the main unit and several tags. A tag is to be attached to each object, such as wallets, bankbook boxes, and smartphones. You can locate the object by pushing the button of the main unit to have the tag emit an alarm. You can find these devices on the Internet with names such as "Locator" or "Finder."
- Make a habit of checking your belongings by pointing to each of them in order to prevent you from leaving them behind when you go out.
- Paste the list of belongings on the back of the entrance door. Check the belongings with the list when you go out. The list also includes the following warnings: "Did I lock the windows?" and "Did I check the gas and fire?"

2. How should I keep a diary and take notes?

- Write a note as soon as you come up with something to remember. Keep a memo-pad in your pocket. Or, hang a memo-pad with a pen around your neck during the day. Further, put a stack of sticky-notes inside it. Sticky-notes should also be put in your wallet and in your smartphone cover. Write memos on the sticky-notes and paste them later on diaries.
- Quit the habit of writing in the diary only at night; it will become more difficult for you to recall events from the morning and the afternoon.
- In order to become accustomed to keeping a diary, set alarms to emit beeps automatically several times a day for writing in the diary.
- Use the New Memory Support Diary or the Diary *Tomorrow* (Yasuda, 2022 *) to prevent forgetfulness. Leave open the diary on your desk and write into it immediately when you think of something you want to remember. Your family members may write in the diary as a message board. You can attach commercialized sticky-notes on each section of the diaries. For example, you could write a schedule on the sticky-notes, and paste it on the "plan" section of the diary.
- When you use an ordinary notebook as the diaries mentioned above, use a double spread page for a day. The page should be divided into sections in advance, such as plan, accounting, meals, and personal belongings. On the blank page of the double-page spread, letters, fliers, photos, receipts should be kept as daily logs.

- If you forget your daily routine, make a "To Do" list every day and check the item when you finish the task. If you copy the list for the day of the week, writing down a "To Do" list for the following weeks will become easy by adding only new errands.
- Use a digital clock with a date display. It may become difficult to identify the date on the normal calendar if dementia progresses.
- When you make an appointment with your friends, inform them of the possibility of your forgetting about it in advance. You may ask them to give you a call or send you an email message to remind you about it.

3. How do I use my smartphone and the IC Recorder?

- Record instructions for taking medicines on your IC Recorder and set the timer to emit recorded instructions. Once you set the timer, the instructions will be played automatically every day, every week, or on the day specified. This function is only supplied by the Sony IC Recorder ICD-PX 240 (Yasuda, 2022 *).
- Set alarms on your smartphone for daily activities such as taking medicine, or charging the phone before you go to bed every night, and wearing your smartphone after you wake up every morning.
- Attach a cord to your smartphone and tie it to a pocket of your clothes with a clip or hang it around your neck. Do not use a stretchable cord to prevent it from dropping into water.
- Use your smartphone every day in order not to forget how to use it. Set up practice times every day. If you have difficulties in using it, remote counseling companies may provide paid services for the operation of smartphones.
- Call your children or friends every morning and let them know how you are doing. Even if they do not pick up your call, they can check the record of your call on their phone.
- Make sure your smartphone has GPS in case of emergency or to prevent getting lost. Ask your remote family members to practice finding you with their smartphones.
- By using an application, such as "LINE," you can record information on it, such as where you put your wallet, what you did, and what you heard, just like filling in the diary. Later, you can search the contents using keywords such as "wallet."
- Record onto your IC Recorder important conversations with your doctors or other professionals at places such as hospitals, banks, and the

city hall. You can confirm the contents later. The IC Recorder is superior for long recordings and has a better sound quality than smartphones.

- When you think of something to do and somewhere to go, such as upstairs or the next room, record your thought on the IC Recorder or a key chain-type recorder immediately before going there. If you cannot recall it, play it back from them.

4. How do I prevent myself from forgetting to take medicines?

- Ask your doctors to prescribe medicines that are to be taken once a day if possible.
- Put medicines on the table before you have each meal.
- In order to prevent taking the same medicine twice, check off the medicine you have just taken on a medicine record chart or in your diary.
- Put the empty packages of medicines temporally in a small box on the table so that you can check if you have already taken them or not.
- Use a calendar (weekly or monthly) with medicine pockets. Electronic medicine boxes (daily, weekly, monthly) can emit alarms at set times.
- Set alarms for the medicine times on your smartphone, the IC Recorder, and others.

5. How do I manage my money and property?

- Store various ID's and passwords for digital properties (cards, devices, onlines, etc.) in one place. Give a copy to a family member.
- Set up automatic payments by bank transfer for water, gas, and electricity.
- Get into the habit of using credit cards or smartphone payments before it becomes difficult for you to handle coins and bills for payments.
- It may become difficult for you to manage your bank accounts if you have many of them. Combine multiple bank accounts to one or reduce the number of accounts in advance.
- Decide the place to keep your bankbooks. Withdraw a small amount of money from your account on the same day of each week. If you withdraw a large amount of money to keep at home, you risk having trouble finding it when you need it.
- Ask your family members to take care of your bankbooks and property at an early stage. Ask them to withdraw a small amount of money from your accounts regularly and to give you a copy of the transactions.
- Keep receipts for money you loaned to or borrowed from your friends,

relatives, and even your spouse and children to prevent you from forgetting about these transactions.

- Put certification documents such as life insurance and real estate contracts together into one folder. Make copies of them and ask your family members to keep the copy.
- Contact the social welfare council in your area for advice on the adult guardianship system as well as banking and property management programs.

6. How do I deal with gas, telephones and appliances?

- Do not use kerosene heaters. Use electric air conditioners for both summer and winter.
- Use a kettle with a whistle or a simple electric pot to boil water.
- Stop using gas stoves and ovens and cook with an IH (Induction Heating) stovetop.
- Change electric lights in the bathroom and in corridors, to ones with a human detection sensor.
- If you have a call or a visitor while using the gas stove, turn off the stove first and then answer the call or go to the door.
- Do not leave the gas stove unattended. When unavoidable, set a timer to alert you to check it.
- Install sensors on gas stoves to prevent overheating without water in pans and pots.
- Make sure to install sensors and alarms to detect abnormal heat, smoke, or gas in the room.
- To cope with fraudulent phone calls, use a telephone that automatically records the conversation. Or use telephones equipped with anti-fraud call functions.
- Set your telephone to respond "please record your message" whenever it receives an incoming call, and answer the phone only when you recognize the caller.
- Attach the remote control for appliances to a table or the wall with cords (or Velcro) to prevent losing them.
- Convert your home appliances into internet-enabled ones that will automatically inform your remote family members when you use them.

7. What else should I do when my forgetfulness has become worse?

- Write statements of your will in the ending note for the possibility that you become bedridden and/or need life-prolonging treatments.

- Inform your friends and neighbors about your forgetfulness and give them brochures explaining about the disease. Ask for their support when necessary.
- When you have hearing impairment, ask an audiologist about hearing aids. Learn how to use them properly at an early stage. The later you begin to use them, the harder it will be to become accustomed to them.
- Do exercises to prevent falls! Use a pedometer, or pedometer application, to motivate yourself to go for a walk. Invite your friends to walk with you. Record the number of steps in your diary.
- Remove electric cords and rugs that make floors uneven in order to prevent falls.
- Organize your photo albums and put titles on each photo. The photos with titles will help you remember important people and events when dementia progresses.
- Someday you may become unable to drive a car. Plan for other means of transportation in advance. You may drive an electric bicycle, an electric tricycle, or a senior car which is set at low speed.
- Use food delivery services. Some companies have their delivery staff members check the user's heath condition at the time of delivery.
- Have conversations with your friends via videophone regularly. Build networks for remote mutual support with your relatives and friends.
- Place personal information cards in a transparent folder and put it in a pocket on your refrigerator. Make a note on the refrigerator door, "My emergency information is in this pocket" in red ink.
- You should also carry this personal information card with you in case of emergency.

* See the following for details: Kiyoshi Yasuda (2022). Rehabilitation for MCI and Dementia: Using Assistive Technology to Support Daily Activities. Or, see the following website of Kiyoshi Yasuda: https://gensoshi.jimdofree.com/homepages-for-english/, or search with "Kiyoshi Yasuda homepage."

Index

FAQs and coping methods

FAQs

Coping methods

Products and applications (app)

Products

Applications (app) of smartphone